General Practitioners Handbook
BRITISH MEDICAL ASSOCIATION

NORMAN ELLIS

Under Secretary, British Medical Association

Foreword by

IAN BOGLE

Chairman, General Medical Services Committee,
British Medical Association

RADCLIFFE MEDICAL PRESS

Radcliffe Medical Press Ltd
18 Marcham Road, Abingdon, Oxon OX14 1AA, UK

Radcliffe Medical Press, Inc.
141 Fifth Avenue, New York, NY 10010, USA

British Library Cataloguing in Publication Data

A catalogue record for this book is available from the British Library.

ISBN 1 85775 241 4

Library of Congress Cataloging-in-Publication Data is available.

Typeset by Advance Typesetting Ltd, Oxfordshire
Printed and bound by Biddles Ltd, Guildford and King's Lynn

Contents

Foreword

A book which explains in clear and concise terms the business side of general practice is long overdue. This book fills the gap. It provides an important reference document for any practice and is particularly relevant to the needs of younger principals, GP registrars and other doctors who have recently entered general practice. Each chapter provides a useful account of a key facet of general practice and tells the reader how to obtain further advice and assistance.

IAN BOGLE
Chairman
General Medical Services Committee
British Medical Association

Preface

This is the first edition of the BMA's *General Practitioners Handbook* which draws heavily upon a previous publication, *Making Sense of General Practice*, edited by Norman Ellis.

The Handbook is directly relevant to both GPs and their practice staff, particularly those who have recently entered into general practice such as GP registrars, newly appointed GP principals and newly appointed staff. While the book brings together factual accounts of several key aspects of the business side of general practice, its overriding aim is to describe clearly and concisely the principles and rules governing the business side of general practice. As the book provides an outline and summary of its various subjects, the reader is told at the beginning of each chapter where to go for further information, advice and assistance.

1 Independent Contractor Status

Where to obtain advice and assistance

GP principals or doctors seeking to become principals can seek the advice of their Local Medical Committee (LMC) secretary. Additionally, BMA members should contact their local BMA offices for expert advice and assistance. Help can also be obtained from Health Authority and LMC offices.

Further reading includes Ellis N and Chisholm J (1997) *Making Sense of the Red Book*. Third edition, Radcliffe Medical Press, Oxford, the Red Book itself and the NHS (General Medical Services) Regulations 1992.

An independent contractor is a self-employed person who has entered into a contract for services with another party. This contract for services is fundamentally different from the contract of service which governs an employee–employer relationship. A key test, often used to distinguish between these two types of contract, relates to the question of 'control'. Generally, the more control A exercises over B's work, the more likely A is to be the employer and B the employee. Thus, if A can tell B not only what job to do but how it is to be done, A has sufficient control to make him B's employer.

However, if the exercise of control is much more diffuse, such that the person doing the work is not told how to do it, the contract is for services and the relationship is between what is confusingly known in legal terminology as 'the principal party' and 'an independent contractor'. Obviously, this test is crude and there are borderline cases, but the status of the National Health Service (NHS) general practitioner (GP) as an independent contractor has not been seriously questioned in the past. As an independent contractor, a GP should not be told by the Health Authority (HA) or Health Board how to practise. HAs and Health Boards should seek to persuade and advise, not direct or control.

British general practice has been strongly influenced by the independent contractor status of its practitioners. The remuneration system, the organization of practices into partnerships, together with the medico-political institutions that enable GPs to exercise professional self-government, illustrate this influence.

As independent contractors, GPs exercise discretion and freedom in how they run their practices. This autonomy carries with it the administrative and financial responsibility for running the business itself and also responsibility for the clinical services provided. These responsibilities include providing premises, staff and equipment. If GPs were employees (like hospital consultants), an NHS Trust or Health Authority would be responsible for providing these resources.

The main advantages of an independent contractor service are its flexibility and adaptability, and its capacity to offer a more personalized model of care. It also provides opportunities for innovation and diversity without interference, and gives patients scope for choice. Disadvantages can arise if the standards of service are allowed to vary widely. Those who are responsible for administering GPs' contracts sometimes see this arrangement as untidy and unsatisfactory, mainly because it lacks the means of control available to an employer.

No other occupation (apart from the other family health services contractor professions – dentists, chemists and opticians) has this unique partnership with the State, or with the public. In current parlance, general practice could be said to be the original 'privatized' sector of the NHS. GPs in other Western developed economies, together with most other professionals, such as dentists, lawyers, architects, surveyors and accountants, are also independent contractors. In Britain, GPs have jealously guarded their independent contractor status ever since Lloyd George's national insurance scheme was introduced in 1913. Although the profession supported the idea of a State-funded medical scheme, it was adamantly opposed to a salaried service; it felt that the loss of independent contractor status would undermine its freedom to practise without State interference and ultimately put patient care at risk. GPs feared that government would seek to direct them in their day-to-day treatment of patients.

The implementation of the 1990 contract has changed the relationship between individual GPs and HAs and Health Boards. New controls are being exercised by HAs and Health Boards over the work of GPs. They are now required to submit an annual report to the HA/Health Boards giving information on their practice arrangements, and also have to provide a detailed statement of the hours they are available to patients for surgery consultations, clinics and home visits.

Additionally, the 1990 contract specifies more precisely which services GPs are required to provide for patients, which procedures should be undertaken and which patients should be offered which services. For example, the terms of service have been amended to make clear that health promotion and illness prevention fall within the remit of general medical services. The services that are required of the GP are spelt out in some detail.

It is perhaps not surprising therefore that, since 1990, the view has gained ground – particularly among younger doctors – that there should be an option for GPs to become salaried employees of the NHS. Salaried status is often seen as a less open-ended commitment than independent contractor status and more in keeping with flexible patterns of employment. The GMSC is committed to ensuring that salaried service is available for those that would prefer it and this view has been reflected in recent policy statements by the Government.

2 How GPs' Pay is Determined

The Doctors' and Dentists' Review Body (DDRB) was set up in 1960, as a consequence of the recommendations of a Royal Commission known as the Pilkington Commission. Its remit is to recommend to the Prime Minister the levels of remuneration of doctors (and dentists) working in the NHS.

The Pilkington Commission was concerned to ensure that doctors' pay should not be used as a means of regulating pay movements in the economy; it wanted to see their pay removed from the political arena. The Commission considered various options, including direct negotiations, collective bargaining through Whitley machinery (used by most health service employees), and arbitration. It finally recommended an independent review body and laid down its ground rules (*see* Box 2.1).

How the Review Body system works

Although the Review Body is willing to receive evidence from any interested party, it concentrates on evidence from a few key sources (*see* Box 2.2). Both sides, the professions and the Health Department, normally submit written evidence to the Review Body on the same day, and also exchange evidence. This means that each side prepares its evidence 'in the dark' without sight of the other's evidence.

The next stage involves oral hearings. The Review Body meets each side, using the occasion to clarify any subject raised in the written evidence or to discuss other points of concern. The parties will also use the oral sessions to emphasize or update any matter in their written evidence.

Having considered all the evidence, the Review Body reports in confidence to the Prime Minister. Further time usually elapses before the

Box 2.1: The Review Body's ground rules as laid down by the Pilkington Commission

- the Review Body's main task was to exercise 'good judgement'
- although the government had the ultimate power to decide, Review Body recommendations must only be rejected by government very rarely, and for most obviously compelling reasons
- government should deal with Review Body recommendations promptly
- the remuneration of doctors should be determined primarily, though not exclusively, by external comparison with other professions and similarly qualified employees
- doctors should not be used by governments as part of their machinery for regulating the economy; they have a right to be treated fairly and the profession should assist the Review Body by willingly providing information about earnings
- doctors' earnings should not be determined according to short-term supply and demand considerations

Box 2.2: Main sources of evidence to the Review Body

- written evidence from the medical profession prepared by the BMA
- written evidence from the dental profession
- written evidence from the Health Department
- joint written evidence agreed between the profession and the Health Department, usually dealing with matters already agreed in negotiation
- jointly agreed statistical information, e.g. evidence on GPs' earnings and expenses
- independent evidence prepared by the Review Body's secretariat (Office of Manpower Economics), e.g. various surveys conducted at the request of the Review Body

report is published and the government announces its decision on whether to implement the recommendations (usually in February).

GPs' remuneration

As independent contractors, GPs are paid a gross income by the NHS, out of which they meet practice expenses, including such items as staff salaries, the cost of surgery premises, and motoring expenses. The GPs' payment system is based on a principle known as 'cost plus'; the payments received are intended both to cover their expenses and to provide a net income (before tax).

The Review Body recommends what it considers to be an appropriate level of net income for GPs, and taking account of this recommendation the government decides upon the average level of income of all GPs. In fact, individual GPs receive greatly varying amounts depending upon the particular circumstances of their practices; expenses and list sizes differ and GPs provide a varying range of services. Virtually all GPs earn either more or less than the average; it is exceptionally rare to discover a GP whose earnings coincide exactly with the average figure.

The component for expenses is added to net income. All expenses incurred by GPs in providing general medical services are paid back to the profession in full: some are paid directly to the individual GP actually incurring them (these are known as directly reimbursed expenses); the remainder of GPs' expenses are reimbursed indirectly on an averaging basis through the fees and allowances. Thus, the exact amount an individual GP receives in indirectly reimbursed expenses will not, except by pure chance, equal expenditure, and in practice, there will be a strong incentive for a GP to economize on his or her own practice expenses.

Although this way of dealing with GPs' expenses is complex and can lead to anomalies and inequalities, it does recognize the independent contractor status of the family doctor, which is fundamentally different from that of salaried doctors employed elsewhere in the NHS. A possible alternative approach could have been to require each GP to submit to the Health Authority or Board a monthly or quarterly claim for expenses, which it would check (and no doubt query on occasion). If this arrangement was adopted, the profession would reduce its independence to choose how to run its practices. The significance of this is not always recognized by those who call for increased direct reimbursement.

It has been argued that because on average a third of any practice's expenses are repaid indirectly through fees and allowances, irrespective of what it actually spends, the less an individual practice spends the greater will be its profits. Although there is some truth in this view, it does not represent the whole picture. GPs are directly reimbursed for part of the cost of providing many of the most costly items (for example, surgery premises and practice staff). A GP who chooses to underfund his or her practice will find it lagging behind other practices in the neighbourhood. A contrary and more positive view needs to be stated. If those GPs who are unwilling to invest in their own practices would overcome their reticence, the profession as a whole would benefit through the indirect reimbursement system and general practice would become more capital intensive. For example, if every GP decided to invest in an ECG machine, under the present system the NHS would have no option but to fund this investment through the indirect reimbursement scheme.

An explanation of how GPs' expenditure on defence body subscriptions is indirectly reimbursed illustrates this point. Almost every GP subscribes to a medical defence body and traditionally the amount each pays has been broadly similar. Thus, every GP is faced with an equivalent level of expenditure. These subscriptions have been paid ever since the present GPs' remuneration structure was established in the 1960s and therefore this expenditure is built into the system. The Review Body is aware that defence body subscriptions must be paid and that these have increased substantially. It is therefore able to make provision for this expenditure in its estimates of GPs' expenses, including an element to take account of anticipated increases in the subscription rate. As almost all GPs pay this subscription, it is reimbursed through fees and allowances (and because future increases have been taken into account) at close to the prevailing rate.

Expenditure that is fully and directly reimbursed

Certain practice expenses are reimbursed directly to each GP. However, while the direct reimbursement is treated as practice income, the expenditure is claimed against income tax. The GP's tax return may be used to calculate those expenses to be reimbursed indirectly through the fees and allowances. Direct reimbursements may be full or partial. Those items reimbursed directly and fully are listed in Box 2.3.

Full direct reimbursement of all of a GP's spending under any heading occurs only when the government or some public agency has direct control over its costs, as is the case with national insurance contributions.

Box 2.3: Items of GP expenditure that are reimbursed directly and fully

- surgery rent and uniform business rate, water rates, water meter installation and charges, and refuse collection charges
- employer's national insurance contributions in respect of GP registrars and some practice staff
- employer's pension contributions in respect of GP registrars and certain approved schemes for practice staff
- net ingredient cost plus VAT of drugs dispensed under the drug tariff

---

Likewise, the GP receives full direct reimbursement of surgery rent if the rent is approved by a district valuer. A GP trainer receives full reimbursement for the registrar's salary and car allowance, and employer's national insurance and superannuation contributions, again because all these costs are within the control of government.

Expenditure that is partially directly reimbursed

The most common partial direct reimbursement is the refund of practice staff salaries. Examples of allowances with maximum or fixed ceilings include those relating to the employment of an assistant, employment of a locum to cover a GP's absence because of sickness, maternity or study leave, and payments made under the doctors' retainer scheme.

The imposition of cash limits on the funds available to Health Authorities and Boards for direct reimbursements means that the percentage of the salary refunded in respect of staff appointments may vary. Health Authorities and Boards can exercise discretion in determining the level of direct reimbursements, and thus it may vary from zero to 100%.

A scheme for the partial direct reimbursement of computing costs was introduced in 1990, and provides for the direct payment of a proportion of the costs of purchasing, leasing, upgrading and maintaining a computer system. More recently, the out of hours development fund established in September 1995 provides for the partial reimbursement of the costs associated with maintaining or improving a high standard of out of hours care.

Indirectly reimbursed expenditure

As described above, each year the Review Body estimates on the basis of a survey of tax returns, how much GPs as a whole will spend on providing general medical services. By taking into account the total Health Authority/Board expenditure on direct reimbursements, it is then able to calculate an average figure for GPs' indirect expenses. This figure for average indirect expenses is added to the level of pre-tax pay which the Review Body considers appropriate for GPs to earn, known as net remuneration, and the resulting figure is called the gross remuneration. The various fees and allowances that comprise a GP's pay are then adjusted so that during the year they yield for the average GP the total gross remuneration which the Review Body has deemed appropriate.

This exercise is complex, and because the 'targets' set by the Review Body are not always met, any under- or over-payment is allowed for in subsequent years. As the Health Department is apprised of how much has been paid to GPs after the end of a financial year, it is not difficult to compare the level of average gross pay received with the Review Body's original target. Average net pay is more difficult to calculate because it depends upon an analysis of income tax returns.

Because GPs wish to obtain tax relief, they inform the Inland Revenue of the expenditure they have incurred in providing general medical services. This is the key source of information for estimating GP expenses. Once a year, the Inland Revenue provides anonymized information relating to a sample of GPs' tax returns, which include professional and partnership expenses.

GP accounts

As the level of expenses to be reimbursed is always based upon samples of income tax returns, it is vital that all GPs record all their expenses correctly.

For revenue items, GPs should enter the full amounts of both directly and indirectly reimbursed expenses, including those items that may not appear in cash books, bank statements or cheque books. Examples include those payments made by Health Authorities and Boards directly to local authorities or other bodies on behalf of the practice, such as health centre rents, waste disposal charges and levies. The practice of 'netting off' expenses against matching income must be avoided; failure to include expenses, however small, has the potential to reduce the funding available to the profession as a whole.

Where capital items are concerned – for example, computers and equipment purchased from the practice fund management allowance – standard accounting practice should be followed. This will usually involve depreciating assets net of any reimbursement received.

3   GPs' Terms of Service

GPs working in the NHS have a contract with the Health Authority or Health Board to provide general medical services for their NHS patients. It is important to note that this contract is with the Health Authority or Health Board and not the patient, in contrast to most other countries where doctors have a direct contractual commitment to patients. Given this independent contractor status with a statutory authority within a publicly funded health service, it is not surprising to find that the NHS GPs' contract has been enshrined in legislation, the NHS (General Medical Services) Regulations (*see* Box 3.1). It is important to bear in mind that as a result of the Government's White Paper, *Primary care: the future – choice and opportunity*, new contractual options may be introduced. New options are expected to be piloted, commencing in 1997.

The regulations, which include the GP's terms of service, provide the legal framework within which the business of NHS general practice is conducted. Because these regulations are laid down by Parliament their style is inevitably legalistic and makes them difficult for a layman to comprehend; a difficulty which is compounded by subsequent amending

---

Box 3.1: National Health Service (General Medical Services) Regulations 1992

The regulations are in seven parts.

I   General: citation and commencement; interpretation; scope and terms of service

II The Medical List: medical list; applying for inclusion or succession to a vacancy; amending of or withdrawing from it; removal from it; local directory of family doctors

III Medical Practices Committee: membership; reports; procedure for filling vacancies; certifying sale of goodwill not involved

IV General Medical Services other than Child Health Surveillance Services, Contraceptive Services, Maternity Medical Services and Minor Surgery Services: describes how patients apply to be on a doctor's list; how patients are assigned to doctors; the limits on list size; how patients transfer to another doctor; how patients are removed from a doctor's list; arrangements for temporary residents; temporary arrangements for running a practice

V   Child Health Surveillance Services, Contraceptive Services, Maternity Medical Services and Minor Surgery Services: explains the separate lists for each of these services and how these services are obtained

VI Payments to doctors: requires the Secretary of State to publish the Statement of Fees and Allowances (the Red Book) and to pay doctors accordingly

VII Miscellaneous: whether a substance is a drug; appointment of medical advisers; guidance to doctors

---

legislation. The regulations have been amended on many occasions; more than a dozen amendments were enacted after 1 April 1985 following the introduction of the limited list of NHS drugs. In November 1989 major amendments were introduced to implement new contractual arrangements with effect from 1 April 1990, and each GP was sent a copy of the amended terms of service. In April 1992 a completely revised and consolidated version of the regulations was made, and a copy of this was also sent to each GP. This new version rationalized the arrangement of the regulations and no longer includes the pharmaceutical services regulations.

Therefore, at the same time as the consolidated General Medical Services Regulations were published, consolidated pharmaceutical services regulations were also distributed. They included regulations governing the provision of pharmaceutical services by doctors, and how rurality is determined in relation to doctor and chemist dispensing.

There is an understandable reluctance to provide a definitive explanatory guide to the regulations. Since they carry the force of law, any dispute about their application or meaning can be resolved only by reference to the original text. Each copy of the regulations, and subsequent amending regulations, is accompanied by an official explanatory note, but it is always stated that this note does not form part of the regulations as such. Nevertheless, a doctor needs to know what is required to fulfil the contract with the Health Authority or Health Board. In part, this knowledge is acquired from colleagues and partners, and the Health Authority/Health Board. Advice from both LMCs and BMA local offices help to familiarize the doctor with the regulations and terms of service. Such advice should help a GP to be aware of current issues concerning their interpretation and application.

Every GP should have access to a copy of the principal regulations and any amending regulations. Copies are distributed by Health Authorities and Health Boards and additional copies may be obtained from them. Nevertheless, many practices rarely refer to the regulations and, if a difficulty ever arises, a GP usually seeks advice from his or her LMC secretary or Health Authority/Health Board general manager.

Alleged breaches of the terms of service by a GP are normally dealt with by the disciplinary committee of a neighbouring Health Authority/Health Board. (The Health Authority/Health Board with which the GP is in contract is a party to the disciplinary proceeding, so its own disciplinary committee cannot conduct the hearing.) A separate set of regulations deals with the MSC procedure, the NHS (Service Committees and Tribunal) Regulations 1992.

It is essential that all GPs are aware of the General Medical Services Regulations because they contain the terms of service which form the basis of their NHS contracts. They should be referred to if any problems arise, and if there is any doubt about their meaning GPs should seek advice from their LMC.

The commentary below focuses on the main aspects of a GP's terms of service; it should help GPs to understand that section of the regulations (an appendix entitled schedule 2) which contains those terms of service. **This selective commentary is not a substitute for the original text and should not be quoted if any problem arises.**

The GP's terms of service

Professional judgement

When a GP has to decide what, if any, professional action needs to be taken under the terms of service, he or she is not expected to exercise a higher degree of skill, knowledge and care than may reasonably be expected of GPs generally. Any GP who wants clarification on a matter involving professional judgement should consult his or her LMC secretary or defence body, or the GMC publication, *Duties of a doctor*. The same general principle also applies to GPs providing child health surveillance or maternity medical or minor surgery services; in each case the level of skill, knowledge and care expected is that which may reasonably be expected of any doctor included in the appropriate list.

Patients

The terms of service specify those categories of persons who are a GP's patients (*see* Box 3.2). Most are self-evident. However, it is important to note that if a patient seeking treatment claims to be on a GP's list but fails to produce a medical card, and the GP has reasonable doubts about the claim, the GP should nevertheless provide treatment but is entitled to ask for a fee. If the patient is subsequently able to prove to the Health Authority or Health Board that he or she is on the GP's list, the fee has to be refunded. In practice, few GPs levy this charge; it is likely to be misunderstood and is rarely worthwhile.

Providing child health surveillance and minor surgery

GPs on the Health Authority or Health Board list may provide to a patient on their list (or on a partner's list or the list of a GP with whom they are in group practice) child health surveillance and/or minor surgery services, and be paid for these services.

A GP who has agreed to provide child health surveillance services should:

- provide those services listed in Box 3.3 below (except for any examination the parent refuses to allow) until the child attains the age of five years
- maintain the records specified in Box 3.4
- provide the health authority with the information specified in Box 3.5.

GPs who have agreed to provide minor surgery services should:

- offer to provide any of the procedures listed in Box 3.6 as appropriate

Box 3.2: Who are a GP's patients?

The main categories are:

- persons on the GP's list
- persons whom the GP has accepted or agreed to accept on the list whether or not the Health Authority or Health Board has received notification of that acceptance
- for a limited period of up to 14 days, persons the GP has refused to accept on to the list, if they live in the practice area and are not on the list of another doctor in the same area, or persons the GP has refused to accept as temporary residents
- persons who have been assigned to the GP under Regulation 21
- for a limited period, persons about whom the GP has been notified that an application has been made for assignment to him or her
- persons accepted as temporary residents
- persons eligible for acceptance as temporary residents whom the GP agrees to take a cervical smear from, vaccinate or immunize
- persons to whom the GP is requested to give treatment which is immediately required owing to an accident or other emergency at any place in the practice area, or any persons to whom the GP agrees on request to give treatment which is immediately required owing to an accident or other emergency at any place in the Health Authority or Health Board locality, provided that there is no other doctor at the time otherwise obliged and available to give treatment
- persons for whom the GP is acting as a deputy to another doctor under the terms of service
- persons whom the GP has been appointed to treat temporarily
- persons for whom the GP has undertaken to provide child health surveillance or minor surgery services
- women for whom the GP has undertaken to provide contraceptive or maternity medical services
- persons whose own doctor has been relieved of responsibility for them during hours arranged with the Health Authority or Health Board, for whom the GP has accepted responsibility during those hours.

Box 3.3: Child health surveillance: services

These services comprise:

- the monitoring:
  (i) by the consideration of information concerning the child received by or on behalf of the doctor, and
  (ii) on any occasion when the child is examined or observed by or on behalf of the doctor (whether pursuant to sub-paragraph (b) or otherwise) of the health, well-being and physical, mental and social development (all of which characteristics are referred to as 'development') of the child while under the age of five years with a view to detecting any deviations from normal development
- the examination of the child by or on behalf of the doctor on so many occasions and at such intervals as shall have been agreed by the Health Authority, or by the Health Board, in whose district the child resides ('the relevant health authority') for the purpose of the provision of child health surveillance services generally in that district.

Box 3.4: Child health surveillance: records

The GP should keep an accurate record of:

- the development of the child under the age of five years, compiled as soon as is reasonably practicable following the first examination and, where appropriate, amended following each subsequent examination, and
- the responses (if any) to offers made to the child's parent for the child to undergo any examination.

Box 3.5: Child health surveillance: information

The GP should provide the health authority with the following information:

- a statement, to be prepared and dispatched to the relevant health authority as soon as is reasonably practicable following any examination, of the procedures undertaken in the course of that examination and of the doctor's findings in relation to each such procedure
- such further information regarding the development of the child while under the age of five years as the relevant health authority may request.

Box 3.6: Minor surgery procedures

Injections	intra-articular
	peri-articular
	varicose veins
	haemorrhoids
Aspirations	joints
	cysts
	bursae
	hydrocele
Incisions	abscesses
	cysts
	thrombosed piles
Excisions	sebaceous cysts
	lipoma
	skin lesions for histology
	intradermal naevi, papillomata, dermatofibromata and similar conditions
	warts
	removal of toe nails (partial or complete)
Curette cautery and cryocautery	warts and verrucae
	other skin lesions (e.g. molluscum contagiosum)
Other	removal of foreign bodies
	nasal cautery

- if providing minor surgery services to a patient not on their list, inform the patient's GP in writing of the outcome of the procedure.

Terminating responsibility for patients

GPs may apply to the Health Authority or Health Board to have a patient removed from their list. This takes effect on the day when the patient is accepted by, or assigned to another doctor, or on the eighth day after applying, whichever is sooner. However, if a GP is treating the person when removal would normally take effect, the Health Authority or Health Board should be informed and removal will take effect only on the eighth day after it receives notification that the patient no longer requires treatment, or upon acceptance by another doctor, whichever occurs first.

From April 1994, GPs may require the Health Authority/Health Board to remove immediately from their list any patient who has given them reasonable cause to fear for their safety, including those who have shown threatening behaviour. The criterion is the GP's reasonable fear. Before immediate removal, the GP *must* inform the police of the incident. This is, in any case, good practice, since a criminal offence under the Public Order or Offences Against the Person Acts will usually have been committed. Having registered the incident with the police, GPs should notify the Health Authority/Health Board of their wish to remove the patient; regardless of whether its offices are open at the time, the removal takes effect from the moment the message reaches the authority. Fax or telephone notification is sufficient, but this should be confirmed in writing. GPs are also required to notify the patient too, but this can be done by post, or via the police, as appropriate.

The right to remove a patient has to be set out against the duty of an Health Authority or Health Board to assign a patient to a GP if the patient is not acceptable on a voluntary basis. In an area served by only one GP this can severely limit a doctor's right to remove a patient.

A GP may agree with a patient to stop providing her with maternity medical services and failing agreement, may apply for permission to terminate the arrangement. The Health Authority or Health Board may agree to this after considering the views of either party and consulting the LMC. If the GP stops providing maternity medical services the patient must be told so that she can make alternative arrangements.

A GP's agreement to provide child health surveillance services may be terminated:

- by either parent or doctor
- if the child has been removed from the doctor's list (or his or her partner's list or that of a doctor with whom he or she is associated in a group practice)
- if the parent fails to respond within 42 days to an invitation to arrange for the child to attend for examination.

Again, the GP should inform the Health Authority or Health Board and, where appropriate, the patient, if he or she no longer intends to provide these services.

Services to patients

GPs are required to provide for their patients all necessary and appropriate personal medical services of the type usually provided by GPs. These should be provided at the practice premises or, if the condition of the patient requires, where the patient was living when accepted as a patient, or elsewhere in the practice area. The GP is not required to visit or treat the patient at any other place, but care has to be taken to ensure that neither the GP nor a member of his or her staff implies there is a willingness to visit at an address outside the practice area. If this should happen, the GP may be bound by a duty to visit.

There is no obligation to provide contraceptive services, child health surveillance services, minor surgery services, or, except in an emergency, maternity medical services, unless the GP has previously agreed to do so.

The doctor should, unless prevented by an emergency, attend and treat any patient who comes for treatment at the places and during the hours approved by the Health Authority or Health Board, other than a patient who attends when an appointment system is in operation and has not made an appointment. In these circumstances the doctor may decline to see the patient during that surgery period, providing the patient's health would not be put at risk and the patient is offered an appointment to attend within a reasonable time. GPs should take all reasonable steps to ensure that a consultation is not so deferred without their knowledge.

The regulations specify in detail certain services which a GP is required to provide which include:

- giving advice, as appropriate, to a patient about the patient's general health, and in particular about diet, exercise, the use of tobacco, the consumption of alcohol and the misuse of drugs and solvents
- offering patients consultations and, where appropriate, physical examinations to identify or reduce the risk of disease or injury
- offering patients, as appropriate, vaccination or immunization against measles, mumps, rubella, pertussis, poliomyelitis, diphtheria and tetanus
- arranging for patients to be referred to other NHS services
- giving advice to enable patients to obtain help from the local authority social services department.

Paragraph 13 of the Terms of Service was amended in February 1995, to secure greater flexibility for GPs as to how they may best meet their out-of-hours responsibility.

The amendments emphasize that GPs themselves are responsible for judging whether or not a consultation is required, on the basis of the information available, and allow them a similar flexibility when deciding what would be the appropriate location for the consultation, whether it is provided by telephone, at the surgery (or some other clinical setting), or at the patient's home, or whether it requires a direct referral to hospital.

Newly registered patients

If a patient has been accepted on to a GP's list (or assigned to it) the patient should be offered a consultation within 28 days to:

- obtain details of the patient's medical history, and when relevant that of his or her family, relating to:
    (i)   illnesses, immunizations, allergies, hereditary conditions, medication and tests carried out for breast or cervical cancer
    (ii) social factors (including employment, housing and family circumstances) which may affect health
    (iii) life-style factors (including diet, exercise, use of tobacco, consumption of alcohol, and misuse of drugs and solvents) which may affect health
    (iv) the current state of the patient's health
- physically examine the patient:
    (i)   measuring height, weight and blood pressure
    (ii) taking and analysing a urine sample to identify the presence of albumin and glucose
- record in the patient's notes the results of this examination
- assess whether and to what extent personal medical services should be provided to the patient
- offer to discuss with the patient (or the parent of a child patient) the conclusions of the consultation as to the state of the patient's health.

When offering a consultation for this purpose, the GP should:

- provide a written invitation – or if the initial invitation is made orally, provide written confirmation
- record in the patient's medical records the date of each invitation and whether it was accepted
- where, as a result of making the invitation, the doctor becomes aware that a patient is no longer residing at the address given in the records, inform the Health Authority or Health Board.

A GP is not required to offer a consultation to a newly registered patient if:

- he or she is a restricted services principal (i.e. a principal who has undertaken to only provide child health services, contraceptive services, maternity medical services, or minor surgery services, or some combination of these)
- the patient is a child under the age of five years
- the patient was, immediately before joining the list, on that of a partner and had already had a consultation of this kind during the previous 12 months.

If a GP assumes responsibility for a list of patients by taking on a vacant practice, or becomes responsible for a sizeable number of new patients over a short period, the GP can ask the Health Authority or Health Board to defer the obligation to offer these consultations.

Patients not seen within three years

If requested to do so, a GP is required to provide to a patient on his or her list a consultation to assess whether personal medical services are needed, if the patient:

- is between the ages of 16 and 75 years
- has within the preceding three years attended neither a consultation with nor a clinic provided by any doctor in the course of the provision of general medical services.

During this consultation the GP should obtain the information listed in Box 3.7 and offer a physical examination including the procedures listed in Box 3.7.

The GP should record the findings and assess whether the patient requires treatment.

Patients aged 75 years and over

The GP should offer each patient an annual consultation and a domiciliary visit (which may be combined) to assess whether any treatment is required. This offer should be made no later than 1 April 1995 to any patient over the age of 75 years on the GP's list on 31 March 1994. For a patient who attains the age of 75 years on or after 1 April 1994, the domiciliary visit and consultation should be offered within 12 months of the patient's 75th birthday. If a patient joins a GP's list and is already aged

Box 3.7: Patients not seen within three years: information to be obtained and procedures to be undertaken during the consultation

Where appropriate the GP should obtain from the patient the following details of his or her medical history and, if relevant to the patient's medical history, that of his or her consanguineous family:

(i)   illnesses, immunizations, allergies, hereditary diseases, medication and tests carried out for breast or cervical cancer

(ii)   social factors (including employment, housing and family circumstances) which may affect health

(iii) life-style factors (including diet, exercise, use of tobacco, consumption of alcohol, and misuse of drugs or solvents) which may affect health, and

(iv)   the current state of the patient's health.

The GP should also offer to undertake a physical examination of the patient, comprising:

(i)   the measurement of blood pressure

(ii)   the taking of a urine sample and its analysis to identify the presence of albumin and glucose, and

(iii) the measurements necessary to detect any changes in body mass;

record in the patient's medical records, the findings arising out of the details supplied by, and any examination of, the patient;

assess whether and, if so, in what manner and to what extent the GP should render personal medical services to the patient; and

in so far as it would not, in the opinion of the doctor, be likely to cause serious damage to the physical or mental health of the patient to do so, offer to discuss with the patient the conclusions the doctor has drawn as a result of the consultation as to the state of the patient's health.

75 years, the offer should be made within 12 months. The GP should make the offer in writing (or confirm it in writing if made orally) and keep a record of the date of the invitation and whether it was accepted.

The doctor should record anything which appears to be affecting the patient's general health, including:

- sensory functions
- mobility
- mental condition
- physical condition including continence
- social and physical environment
- use of medicines.

The GP should also record the findings of the consultation and offer to discuss with the patient any conclusions that have been drawn.

Absences, deputies, assistants and partners

Normally, a GP should give treatment personally. However in the case of general medical services, other than maternity medical services, child health surveillance and minor surgery services, the GP is under no obligation to do so if reasonable steps are taken to ensure continuity of treatment by another doctor acting as a deputy, irrespective of whether the other doctor is a partner or an assistant. In addition, if it is reasonable to delegate the clinical treatment to a person whom the GP has authorized and who is competent to carry it out (e.g. a qualified nurse), the GP may do so.

A doctor on the obstetric list should not, without the Health Authority's or Health Board's consent, employ a deputy or assistant to provide maternity services who is not (or is not qualified by experience to be) included on the obstetric list, except in an obstetric emergency.

As for child health surveillance services, a GP who has agreed to provide these may employ a deputy or an assistant on a child health surveillance list, or with the Health Authority's or Health Board's agreement another deputy or assistant. A GP who has agreed to provide minor surgery services may employ a deputy or assistant who is on a minor surgery list.

In general, GPs are responsible for the acts and omissions of any doctors acting as their deputies, whether the deputy is a partner or an assistant. They are similarly responsible for any person they employ or who acts on their behalf. *However, a GP is not responsible under the terms of service for the acts and omissions of a deputy who is on the list of the same or some other Health Authority/Health Board.*

The Health Authority/Health Board should be informed of any stand-ing deputizing arrangements unless the deputy is the GP's assistant or is already on its medical list, and carries out these arrangements at the premises where the doctor normally practises. If a GP is absent for more than a week, the Health Authority/Health Board should be told who is responsible for the practice during their absence.

Before entering into any arrangement with a deputizing service, GPs should obtain the Health Authority's or Health Board's consent. When giving consent, it may impose conditions to ensure that the arrangements are adequate, but must consult the LMC before refusing consent or impos-ing conditions. The Health Authority/Health Board is required to review any consent given or conditions imposed in consultation with the LMC, and may withdraw consent or alter the conditions. A GP may appeal to the Secretary of State against a refusal or withdrawal of consent, or the imposition or variation of conditions.

GPs should take reasonable steps to satisfy themselves that any doctor employed as a deputy or assistant is not disqualified from inclusion on the Health Authority's/Health Board's list. The GP should tell the Health Authority/Health Board the name of any assistant employed and when this employment ends. A doctor should not employ one or more assistants for more than three months in a period of 12 months without its consent, but before refusing or withdrawing consent, it must consult the LMC. (A GP may appeal to the Medical Practices Committee (MPC) against re-fusal or withdrawal of consent.) If consent is withdrawn, the decision will not take effect for a month; but if an appeal is made to the MPC against withdrawal and it dismisses the appeal, the withdrawal takes effect from a date determined by the MPC, not less than one month after the date of dismissal. (A doctor acting as a deputy can treat patients at places and times other than those arranged by the GP for whom he or she is deputiz-ing although regard must be given to the convenience of the patients.)

Arrangements at practice premises

The GP should provide adequate accommodation at the practice premises having regard to the practice's circumstances or any other premises at which the Health Authority/Health Board has agreed (s)he may treat his/her patients, and is required, on receiving a written request from the Health Authority or Health Board, to allow the premises to be visited at any reasonable time by a representative of either the Health Authority/ Health Board or LMC, or both.

If a GP intends to run an appointment system (or succeeds to or joins a practice where one is already running), the Health Authority/Health

---

Box 3.8: Transfer of out of hours responsibility

An extra paragraph (18A) was added to the terms of service in April 1996 to allow GPs to transfer their out of hours responsibility, full or in part, to another GP on a Health Authority/Health Board list. GPs must apply to their Health Authorities/Health Boards for approval for such a transfer of responsibility. Health Authorities/Health Boards should only withhold approval in exceptional circumstances and after consulting the LMC. Paragraph 18A(7) sets out the information which GPs should include in their applications.

Board should be told about the proposed system or of any proposal to discontinue it.

With certain important exceptions, a GP should not, without the consent of the Health Authority/Health Board (or, on appeal, the MPC), start to practise in any premises within one year of their having ceased to be occupied or used for practice purposes by another doctor who within one month of such cessation begins practising at a group practice premises, as a member of a group, or at a health centre less than three miles away from the original premises. (This does not apply if the former occupant gives written consent for another doctor to use the premises.)

Employees

Before employing any member of staff, the GP should ensure that the person is suitably qualified and competent to carry out the required duties. In particular, the doctor should take account of the employee's academic and vocational qualifications, training and previous experience. The GP should also offer the employee reasonable training opportunities.

Availability to patients

Any GP should normally be available at times and places approved by the Health Authority/Health Board and inform patients of his or her availability. In general, it will not approve any application unless satisfied that the times proposed are such that the GP is normally available:

- 42 weeks in any period of 12 months
- during not less than 26 hours in any such week

- on five days in any such week
- with hours of availability which are likely to be convenient to patients.

There are important exceptions to this basic requirement:

- a GP may seek to be normally available for 26 hours over a four-day week, if involved in health-related activities other than providing general medical services to his or her patients (*see* Box 3.9 below, for a broad definition of health related activities). But the four-day availability will not be approved by the Health Authority/Health Board if it considers that the effectiveness of the doctor's services to patients is likely to be significantly reduced or patients are likely to suffer significant inconvenience
- a GP may seek to be available for less than 26 hours a week, if practising in a partnership. In this case there are two options:
  (i) less than 26 hours but not less than 19 hours
  (ii) less than 19 hours but not less than 13 hours
- two doctors in partnership may apply for Health Authority/Health Board approval to be jointly available for 26 hours a week.

Box 3.9: List of health-related activities

- activities connected with the organization or training of the medical profession
- activities connected with the provision of medical care or treatment
- activities connected with the improvement of the quality of such care or treatment
- activities connected with the administration of general medical services
- appointments concerning medical education or training
- medical appointments within the health service other than in relation to the provision of general medical services
- medical appointments under the Crown, with government departments or agencies, or public or local authorities
- appointments concerning the regulation of the medical profession or services on the MPC
- membership of a medical audit advisory group

The NHS Executive has issued important guidance to Health Authorities on the availability requirements of the 1990 contract.

Strictly speaking, under the regulations the availability in question has to be looked at on the basis of each individual doctor's application in respect of his or her hours and their convenience to patients. The regulations do not require Health Authorities to take partners' availability into account, but nor do they preclude them from doing so except in circumstances where:

- this would result in arrangements which were not convenient to the GP's own patients;

OR

- the GP whose application is being considered objects.

The Health Department's view is that, provided these circumstances do not apply, Health Authorities may take account of partnership availability. Appeals made against their decisions on availability have highlighted several areas of uncertainty. The most common of these are summarized below.

- Health Authorities *cannot* stipulate which specific days doctors must be available. Under the regulations it is for doctors to choose which days they wish to be available. The 'convenience to patients' rule then applies to the spread of the hours across the doctor's chosen days. They may not, for example, require a doctor to provide a surgery on a Saturday, if that doctor is already available on five other days each week.

- Many Health Authorities have agreed local policies as to how they deal with applications by doctors for approval of hours of availability. Nevertheless, each application has to be considered individually against the requirements of the terms of service. They may not hold that a doctor's proposed hours are inconvenient merely because they do not meet local criteria. There must be a recognized procedure for looking at each doctor's individual circumstances and convenience to patients.

- The regulations do not specifically require doctors to work the *same* five days every week. There is therefore no bar on doctors working a rota system provided that it meets the 'convenience to patients' test; for example, a fixed and regular rota, which is easily understandable by, and is advertised to, patients.

- Health Authorities have the authority, when approving a doctor's hours of availability, to make its approval subject to specified conditions. However, one such condition may *not* be that approval is limited to a certain period (e.g. approving the hours subject to a review in six months). Any conditions laid down must involve an amendment to the proposed hours of availability which, if accepted by the GP, would result in the hours being agreed.

- Health Authorities do not have the authority to designate a doctor, who has applied on the basis of full-time availability, as a part-time doctor and to reduce rates of pay accordingly. They may *only* reduce rates of payment to those appropriate for GPs working part-time, where it is a condition imposed by the MPC that the doctor should work part-time.

- In the case of doctors applying for four-day availability it is not necessary for the 'health-related activities' concerned to be performed on the day for which relief is being sought. Provided these activities are on a fixed and regular basis, a doctor may be entitled to apply for reduced availability on the basis of the cumulative effects of such activities.

Practice area

A doctor may not open premises in an area where, at the time of the application, the MPC considers the number of GPs to be adequate. Subject to this condition, a GP may apply at any time to the Health Authority for consent to alter the practice area. (If it refuses consent, the GP may appeal to the Secretary of State.)

Notification of change of residence

If a GP changes his or her place of residence, the Health Authority/Health Board should be told in writing within 28 days.

Records

A GP should keep adequate records of the illnesses and treatment of patients on forms supplied by the Health Authority/Health Board, and should send these to it on request as soon as possible. Within 14 days of being informed by the Health Authority of a patient's death (or not later than one month after otherwise learning of it), a GP should return the records to the Health Authority/Health Board.

Certification

A GP should issue to patients or their personal representatives free of charge the certificates listed in Box 3.10 if they are reasonably required.

Box 3.10: List of prescribed medical certificates

Purpose of certificate	*Relevant legislation*
1. To claim payment; to prove inability to work or incapacity, and to draw pensions etc.	Naval and Marine Pay and Pensions Act 1865 Air Force (Constitution) Act 1917 Pensions (Navy, Army, Air Force and Mercantile Marine) Act 1939 Personal Injuries (Emergency Provisions) Act 1939 Pensions (Mercantile Marine) Act 1942 Polish Resettlement Act 1947 Home Guard Act 1951 Social Security Act 1975 Industrial Injuries and Diseases (Old Cases) Act 1975 Parts I and III of the Social Security and Housing Benefits Act 1982 Parts II and V of, and Schedule 4 to, the Social Security Act 1986
2. To prove pregnancy so as to obtain welfare foods	Section 13 of the Social Security Act (1988)
3. To show fitness for inhaling analgesia in childbirth	Nurses, Midwives and Health Visitors Act 1979
4. To register a still-birth	Births and Deaths Registration Act 1953
5. To enable payment to be made to an institution or other person in case of mental disorder of persons entitled to payment from public funds	Section 142 of the Mental Health Act 1983
6. To prove unfitness for jury service	Juries Act 1974

continued overleaf

Box 3.10: *continued*

Purpose of certificate	*Relevant legislation*
7. To prove unfitness for medical examination	National Service Act 1948
8. To support late application for reinstatement in civil employment or notification of non-availability, owing to sickness	Reinstatement in Civil Employment Act 1944 Reinstatement in Civil Employment Act 1950 Reserve Forces Act 1980
9. To register as an absent voter on grounds of physical incapacity	Representation of the People Act 1983
10. To apply for exemption from charges for drugs, medicines and appliances	National Health Service Act 1977
11. To support a severely mentally impaired person's claim for exemption from paying the community charge	Local Government Finance Act 1988
12. To support a claim by or on behalf of a severely mentally impaired person for exemption from liability to pay the Council Tax or eligibility for a discount in respect of the amount of Council Tax payable	Local Government Finance Act 1992

However, a GP is not obliged to do so if the patient is being attended by another doctor (other than a partner, assistant or deputy) or is not being treated by, or under the supervision of, a doctor. In certain circumstances, a GP may issue a statement, without an examination, advising the patient to refrain from work for a period of up to a month, provided a written report, not more than a month old, has been received from another doctor at a hospital, place of employment or other institution. The other doctor should not be a partner, assistant or deputy.

Accepting fees

A GP must not demand or accept a fee or any other form of remuneration for any treatment, including maternity medical services, whether under the terms of service or not, given to a person for whose treatment he or she is responsible. Doctors must take all practical steps to ensure that any partner, deputy or assistant does not demand or accept any remuneration for treatment given to their patients unless, of course, the partner, deputy or assistant would have been entitled to charge if the patient had been on his or her own list.

There are, however, certain specific circumstances in which a GP may accept a fee. These are listed in Box 3.11.

Box 3.11: Specific circumstances in which a GP may accept a fee

- from any statutory body for services rendered for the purpose of that body's statutory functions
- from any body, employer or school for a routine medical examination of persons for whose welfare the body, employer or school is responsible, or an examination of such persons for the purpose of advising the body, employer or school of any administrative action they might take
- for treatment which is not of a type usually provided by GPs and which is given:
  (i) pursuant to the provisions of section 65 of the Act, or
  (ii) in a registered nursing home which is not providing services under the Act
  if, in either case, the doctor is serving on the staff of a hospital providing services under the Act as a specialist providing treatment of the kind the patient requires and if, within seven days of giving the treatment, the doctor supplies the HA, on a form provided by it for the purpose, with such information about the treatment as it may require
- under Section 158 of the Road Traffic Act 1988
- from a dentist in respect of the provision at his request of an anaesthetic for a person for whom the dentist is providing general dental services

continued overleaf

Box 3.11: *continued*

- when he or she treats a patient under paragraph 4(3), in which case he or she shall be entitled to demand and accept a reasonable fee (recoverable under paragraph 39) for any treatment given, if he or she gives the patient a receipt on a form supplied by the Health Authority
- for attending and examining (but not otherwise treating) a patient at his request at a police station in connection with proceedings which the police are minded to bring against him
- for treatment consisting of an immunization for which no remuneration is payable by the Health Authority in pursuance of the Statement made under regulation 34 and which is requested in connection with travel abroad
- for circumcising a patient for whom such an operation is requested on religious grounds and is not needed on any medical ground
- for prescribing or providing drugs which a patient requires to have in his possession solely in anticipation of the onset of an ailment while he is outside the United Kingdom but for which he is not requiring treatment when the medicine is prescribed
- for a medical examination to enable a decision to be made whether or not it is inadvisable on medical grounds for a person to wear a seat belt
- where the person is not one to whom any of paragraphs (a), (b) or (c) of section 38(1) of the Act applies (including by reason of regulations under section 38(6) of that Act), for testing the sight of that person
- where he or she is a doctor who is authorized or required by a Health Authority under regulation 20 of the Pharmaceutical Regulations to provide drugs, medicines or appliances to a patient and provides for that patient, otherwise than under pharmaceutical services, any Scheduled drug
- pursuant to an arrangement with him or her for the provision of services in accordance with Regulation 23 of the NHS (Fundholding Practices) Regulations 1993
- for prescribing or providing drugs for malaria chemoprophylaxis

There are other certificates and reports which are not part of a GP's NHS obligations to patients. Fees for these are a matter to be agreed between the GP and the person or organization requesting the certificate or report; the BMA suggests fees for these procedures.

A doctor must not demand or accept a fee or other remuneration from a patient for prescribing or supplying any drug or chemical reagent or appliance, unless the patient requires it solely in anticipation of the onset of an ailment outside the United Kingdom for which he or she is not currently being treated.

Prescribing and dispensing

A GP is required to supply drugs or listed appliances needed for a patient's immediate treatment before a supply can be obtained elsewhere. In the course of treating a patient under general medical services, a GP must not issue a prescription for a drug or other substance listed in schedule 10 to the regulations (the 'black list') for supply under the NHS. In the case of a drug listed under schedule 11 to the regulations, a doctor may prescribe only in certain circumstances. A GP may prescribe these items privately, but may not charge for doing so. The GP can only charge for the item itself if he or she is already entitled to dispense to a patient and the GP can only do so for a particular course of treatment.

Practice leaflets

A GP or partnership should prepare a practice leaflet including the information in Box 3.12.

The leaflet should be reviewed at least annually to maintain accuracy and an up-to-date copy should be made available to the Health Authority

---

Box 3.12: Information to be included in practice leaflets

Personal and professional details of the doctor:

- full name
- sex
- medical qualifications registered by the General Medical Council
- date and place of first registration as medical practitioner.

continued overleaf

Box 3.12: *continued*

Practice information:

- the times approved by the Health Authority/Health Board during which the doctor is personally available for consultation by his patients at his practice premises

- whether an appointments system is operated by the doctor for consultations at his practice premises

- if there is an appointments system, the method of obtaining a non-urgent appointment and the method of obtaining an urgent appointment

- the method of obtaining a non-urgent domiciliary visit and the method of obtaining an urgent domiciliary visit

- the doctor's arrangements for providing personal medical services when he is not personally available

- the name and address of any other doctor to whom the doctor has made an out of hours arrangement under paragraph 18(A) of the terms of service; also his or her availability times and contact details

- the method by which patients are to obtain repeat prescriptions from the doctor

- if the doctor's practice is a dispensing practice, the arrangements for dispensing prescriptions

- if the doctor provides clinics for his patients, their frequency, duration and purpose

- the numbers of staff, other than doctors, assisting the doctor in his practice, and a description of their roles

- whether the doctor provides maternity medical services, contraceptive services, child health surveillance services or minor surgery services

- whether the doctor works single-handed, in partnership, part-time or on a job-sharing basis, or within a group practice

- the nature of any arrangements whereby the doctor or his staff receive patients' comments on his provision of general medical services

- the geographical boundary of his practice area by reference to a sketch, diagram or plan

continued opposite

Box 3.12: *continued*

- whether the doctor's practice premises have suitable access for all disabled patients and, if not, the reasons why they are unsuitable for particular types of disability
- if an assistant is employed, details for him as specified in paragraphs 1–5 of this table
- if the practice either is a GP training practice for the purposes of the NHS (Vocational Training) Regulations 1979 or undertakes the teaching of undergraduate medical students, and the nature of arrangements for drawing this to the attention of patients.

or Health Board, each patient on the doctor's list and anyone who reasonably requires one.

Complaints

In April 1996 a new NHS procedure for handling complaints about GPs was introduced. A new disciplinary system was also implemented at this time, which is separate from the complaints procedure. New paragraphs were added to the terms of service requiring GPs to:

- establish and operate practice based procedures for dealing with complaints
- cooperate with investigation of complaints by Health Authorities/ Health Boards (this may occur if a complainant is not satisfied with the outcome of a practice based investigation).

Inquiries about prescriptions and referrals

The GP should be prepared to answer any inquiries from the Health Authority or Health Board relating to:

- any prescriptions issued
- referrals to other NHS services.

Annual reports

A GP or partnership should provide the Health Authority or Health Board annually with a report containing the information in Box 3.13. The

Box 3.13: Information to be provided in annual reports

1 particulars of the doctor's other commitments as a medical practitioner, including:

   (a) a description of any posts held, and

   (b) a description of all work undertaken

and including, in each case, the annual hourly commitment, except that where a doctor has notified the Health Authority/ Health Board of such other commitments in a previous annual report, the report need only contain information relating to any changes in those commitments

2 as respects orders for drugs and appliances, the doctor's arrangements for the issue of repeat prescriptions to patients

3 information relating to the referral of patients to other services under the Act during the period of the report:

   (a) as respects those by the doctor to specialists:

      (i) the total number of patients referred as in-patients

      (ii) the total number of patients referred as out-patients

by reference in each case to which clinical specialty applies, and specifying in each case the name of the hospital concerned; and

   (b) the total number of cases of which the doctor is aware (by reference to the clinical specialty) in which a patient referred himself to services under the Act

4 information relating to the numbers of patients on the doctor's list:

   (a) who are diabetic

   (b) who are asthmatic, and

   (c) to whom the doctor has given advice, in accordance with paragraph 12(2) of schedule 2, about:

      (i) the patient's weight

      (ii) the use of tobacco, or

      (iii) the consumption of alcohol

5 number of complaints received under the practice-based procedure.

information in paragraph 3 of the table only needs to be supplied if the Health Authority/Health Board requests it, having considered whether the information is available from another source and having consulted the LMC. The information in paragraph 4 of the table need only be supplied if the Health Authority/Health Board requests it and if the GP is not supplying the information already in order to qualify for health promotion or disease management payments. Each report should be compiled for a 12-month period ending 31 March and should be sent to the Health Authority by 30 June.

Conclusion

This commentary is selective, not comprehensive. Not all paragraphs in the terms of service have been covered and only a brief summary of those referred to has been provided. If any problem arises, a GP should refer to the regulations and if necessary seek the advice and assistance of the LMC secretary or BMA local office.

4 Fees and Allowances

Where to obtain advice and assistance

Help can be obtained from the Health Authority/Board and LMC offices. BMA members can also contact their local BMA office for advice and assistance.

Further reading includes Ellis N and Chisholm J (1997) *Making Sense of the Red Book*. Third edition, Radcliffe Medical Press.

The GPs' pay system is particularly complex and hard to understand. GPs earn their income from a range of fees and allowances. These are of four broad types: fixed allowances, capitation-based payments, item-of-service payments and bonus payments. They are set each year at levels which will both yield the finite 'pool' of money available to fund GPs' net income and meet those expenses not reimbursed directly by the Health Authority or Health Board. The 'pool' which funds GPs' net income is calculated by multiplying average intended net remuneration by the number of GP principals.

If the relative level of any fee or allowance is altered (e.g. by increasing the basic practice allowance or decreasing capitation fees), the remaining fees and allowances are changed so that the total amount of money paid out to GPs remains at the right level. Unless additional funds are specifically made available by government (colloquially known as 'new money'), according to the current pay system it is not possible to increase any specific fees or allowances without simultaneously reducing some other fee(s) so as to maintain the level of net remuneration.

This chapter outlines the main fees and allowances payable to GPs which were newly introduced or substantially modified by the 1990 contract and subsequent additions. Full details of all fees and allowances are given in the Statement of Fees and Allowances (otherwise known as the SFA or Red Book).

Basic practice allowance

GPs qualify for the basic practice allowance (BPA) if their individual list size or partnership average list size is at least 400 patients; a GP with at least 400 patients is paid a BPA and its level increases with list size up to a ceiling of 1200 patients. Thus a lump sum is paid for the first 400 patients and additional capitation payments are then made for each patient between 400 and 600, 600 and 800, 800 and 1000, and 1000 and 1200. By weighting the level of these capitation payments in favour of the lower list size, the BPA is designed to compensate for the proportionately greater standing expenses incurred by a small practice than a larger one. The BPA is also weighted in favour of part-time GPs; that of a half-time GP is significantly greater than half that of a full-time GP.

Deprivation payments

GPs are paid a capitation based supplement to the BPA, known as the 'deprivation payment', for all patients living within an area classified as 'deprived' according to the Jarman deprivation index, whether or not the individual or family is actually deprived. This supplement is intended to reflect the higher workload associated with some categories of patients. GPs with individual or average partnership lists of less than 400 patients who are not paid a BPA, nevertheless qualify for deprivation payments for patients living in deprived areas. There are three levels of payment according to the degree of deprivation (as measured by the Jarman index) of the area where the patient lives.

Seniority payments

There are three levels of seniority payment:
- the first level is paid to a GP registered for 11 years or more and providing general medical services for at least 7 years
- the second level is paid to a GP registered for 18 years or more and providing general medical services for at least 14 years
- the third level is paid to a GP registered for 25 years or more and providing general medical services for at least 21 years.

Pro rata payments are made to part-time GPs and those full-time GPs not eligible for the full BPA. Job-sharers are assessed for the seniority payment on an individual basis and payment is reduced pro rata according to their hours of availability.

Capitation fees

The standard capitation fees are paid at three rates according to a patient's age: under 65 years, 65–74 years, and 75 years and over.

Registration fee

This is paid to a GP who carries out certain health checks on a newly registered patient (except those aged under five years), normally within three months of joining the list.

Postgraduate education allowance

The postgraduate education allowance (PGEA) is paid to any GP who undertakes a programme of continuing education; it is intended to cover any course fees, travel and subsistence costs.

To receive the full rate of the PGEA, GPs must demonstrate to their Health Authority/Health Board that they have attended an average of five days training a year over the past five years. Although the amount of time spent on courses may vary from year to year, a GP is expected to achieve a reasonable balance between years. Courses are divided into three areas:

- health promotion and prevention of illness
- disease management
- service management.

To claim the PGEA, GPs have to attend at least two courses under each of the three subject areas over the five years preceding the claim. The length of course is not actually defined in the Red Book; postgraduate deans have discretion to determine what constitutes a 'course' for the purpose of completing a balanced educational programme.

A GP should claim the allowance from the Health Authority/Health Board each year, giving details of courses attended over the five-year period.

Any GP who meets the required criteria (25 days training and at least two courses under each of the three headings) is paid a full PGEA in quarterly instalments. Lower levels of the allowance are paid if courses are spread across only one or two of the subject areas or less than the maximum length of training is undertaken.

Target payments for childhood immunization and cervical cytology

In 1990 the Government introduced target payments for childhood immunization and cervical cytology. There are two levels of payment. For childhood immunization, a higher level of payment is made to GPs who achieve 90% coverage and a lower level for 70% coverage. For cervical cancer screening the upper level is 80% and the lower 50%. These are calculated on a partnership basis.

Childhood immunization

There are two target levels, 70% and 90%, and these relate to average coverage levels across four groups of immunizations:

- Group I   – diphtheria, tetanus and poliomyelitis
- Group II   – pertussis
- Group III   – mumps, measles and rubella (MMR)
- Group IV   – haemophilius influenzae type B (Hib).

A target is reached if, on average across the four groups, 70% or 90% of the children aged two years on a GP's list have had complete courses of immunization (i.e. three doses of diphtheria, tetanus and poliomyelitis, or three doses of pertussis, or one dose of MMR, or three doses of Hib). To calculate this, the coverage level in each group is taken into account and the mean of these is the overall coverage level. For example, if a practice has 10 children on the list aged two years all of whom have had complete courses of diphtheria, tetanus, poliomyelitis and Hib, nine who have had a complete course of pertussis and eight who have had the MMR immunization, the overall coverage level is nine out of 10, that is 90%. Thus, the higher target level has been reached. All complete immunization courses count towards coverage levels whether done by the GP making the claim or some other person, such as a community health clinic doctor.

The maximum payment a GP can receive depends on how many children aged two years are on the list; the Red Book describes how this is calculated. The proportion of the maximum payment made to a GP reflects the amount of this work done within general medical services, rather than in a clinic or hospital setting, whether in the patient's current practice or a previous one. Thus, if the 90% level is achieved, and GPs have done 70% of all the complete courses of immunization, the claiming GP receives 7/9 of the maximum payment.

Pre-school boosters for children under five years

Again, there are two target levels: 70% and 90%. A target is reached if at least 70% or 90% of children aged five years on a GP's list have had reinforcing doses of diphtheria, tetanus and poliomyelitis immunizations. The arrangements for calculating these payments are similar to those described above.

Cervical cytology

There are two target levels: 50% and 80%; a target is reached if 50% or 80% of women on a GP's list aged 25–64 years in England and Wales (or aged 21–60 years in Scotland) have had an adequate cervical smear test during the previous five-and-a-half years. (This period is based on a five-year call/recall system with an allowance for unavoidable delays.) All smear tests are counted, not just those taken in general practice. For the purpose of calculating coverage, women who have had hysterectomies (involving the complete removal of the cervix) are excluded.

The maximum size of the target payment a GP can receive depends on the number of eligible women on the list. The actual proportion of the maximum payment paid to a GP reflects the work done by GPs (and their staff) as opposed to others, such as the private sector and community health services.

Child health surveillance fee

To be paid for child health surveillance GPs must be on the Health Authority/Health Board child health surveillance list; admission to this requires them to satisfy the criteria relating to experience and training set out in the regulations. A capitation supplement is paid for each child patient under the age of five years to whom a GP provides developmental surveillance, if the child is registered with the GP for this purpose.

Minor surgery payments

A sessional payment is made to GPs on the Health Authority/Health Board minor surgery list who personally provide minor surgery services. A session consists of at least five surgical procedures, performed either in a single clinic or on separate occasions. GPs can undertake minor surgery for patients on their own personal list or that of a partner or another member of the group practice. A GP is eligible for no more than three such payments in respect of any one quarter. However, a GP who is in a partnership or group may claim additional payments, provided the total number of payments to the partnership or group per quarter does not exceed three times the number of GPs involved. Up to four minor surgery procedures can be carried forward for inclusion in the following quarter's claim.

Night fees consultation and night allowance

All GPs are paid an annual night allowance in partial recognition of their 24 hour responsibility for patients. This allowance is paid at a flat rate per GP with job sharers counting as a single GP for this purpose.

In addition GPs are paid a fee for each face to face consultation requested and undertaken between 10 p.m. and 8 a.m. with a patient who is:

- on their list of patients
- a temporary resident
- a woman for whom they had undertaken to provide maternity medical services in connection with which the consultation is provided.

Where the GP is separately engaged or employed by an NHS Trust or Health Authority to provide services in any premises owned or managed by the Trust or Authority, the fee is paid only if the GP is not on duty or on call at those premises and the request for the patient to be seen was made in accordance with paragraph 13 of the terms of service. However, if the GP visits the patient in a hospital to provide maternity medical services, a consultation fee is paid if he or she holds an appointment at the hospital, but was not on duty at the time, or if he or she does not hold such an appointment in respect of maternity medical services.

The fee is paid to the GP with whom the patient is registered, regardless of whether the visit is made by:

- the GP with whom the patient is registered
- a partner or another GP from the practice

- an assistant, associate, GP Registrar, locum or deputy employed by the partnership or group, or a doctor in the same out of hours rota.

Associate allowance

Single-handed GPs in very isolated areas (e.g. the Highlands and Islands) are eligible for an associate allowance, enabling them, in conjunction with other single-handed GPs, to employ an associate GP who can provide services for patients during absences for social and professional purposes.

Health promotion payments

A new payment system based on practices developing their own health promotion programmes was introduced in October 1996. The new scheme is based on a single level of payment for health promotion activities approved by local, professionally led, health promotion committees. The amount a practice receives is related to list size.

Activities must relate to:

- modern authoritative medical opinion
- the Health of the Nation strategy and/or
- patient needs and/or
- local health priorities.

There are separate payments for organizing chronic disease management programmes for either asthma or diabetes. These require practices to develop guidelines for delivering care to these patients.

Other fees and allowances

- additions to the BPA for employing an assistant
- inducement payments
- initial practice allowances
- mileage payments
- temporary resident fees
- fees for emergency treatment

- fees for immediately necessary treatment
- fees for maternity medical services
- fees for contraceptive services
- fees for public policy vaccinations and immunizations
- fees for service as an anaesthetist and for arresting a dental haemorrhage
- payments for supplying drugs and appliances
- payments during sickness and confinement – there are no list size restrictions for employing a locum during confinement
- locum allowances for single-handed practitioners in rural areas attending educational courses
- prolonged study leave allowance
- trainee practitioner scheme payments
- doctors' retainer scheme payments
- payments under the rent and rates scheme
- improvement grants
- payments under the practice staff scheme
- payments under the computer reimbursement scheme.

Claiming correct fees and allowances

The NHS GPs' remuneration system is probably the most complex in the world. It takes several hundred pages and an estimated 350 000 words of the regulations and the Red Book to determine how and what a GP should be paid. Every practice should ensure that it is claiming correct fees and allowances, otherwise it will not receive its correct remuneration. Conversely, no claim should ever be made, whether knowingly or unknowingly, for a fee or allowance to which a GP or practice is not entitled. False or improper claims can have very serious consequences; Health Authorities have not hesitated to instigate criminal proceedings against GPs who have made these.

5 The Partnership Agreement

Where to obtain advice and assistance

BMA members should contact their local BMA office for general advice and assistance. Members can obtain free of charge an authoritative booklet entitled *Medical Partnerships under the NHS*. Health Authorities, Health Boards and LMCs are also important sources of advice. However, both partners and prospective partners should also obtain independent legal advice when entering or substantially amending a partnership agreement, preferably from solicitors who are familiar with medical partnerships.

Further reading includes Ellis N and Stanton T (eds) (1994) *Making Sense of Partnerships*. Radcliffe Medical Press, Oxford.

The partnership provides a legal framework within which most GPs work: less than 10% of practices are single-handed. Given its importance to the business of general practice, the widespread ignorance and neglect of the partnership agreement among the profession is quite remarkable.

Many practices do not have written partnership agreements; it has been estimated that at least half either have no written agreement or work to an outdated version. Any partnership without this essential documentation is susceptible to the vagaries that flow from the fact that relations between the partners are strictly controlled by a century old statute, the Partnership Act 1890. A partnership without a written agreement is known as a 'partnership at will' and is governed by this Act; its main characteristics are listed in Box 5.1. However, a partnership can develop or agree to abide by rules which modify or add to those drawn from this legislation. Variations and departures from the Partnership Act can be inferred from the conduct of the partners; for example, although the Act requires profits to be shared equally, many practices opt for a different basis of division.

Given the dangers and potential difficulties of a 'partnership at will', it is surprising how many practices do not have written agreements. But neglect of essential paperwork has been commonplace in general practice; until comparatively recently most practice staff did not have written employment contracts, even though they were legally entitled to them.

Box 5.1: Key characteristics of a 'partnership at will': one without a written agreement

- entire partnership ends automatically upon death, retirement or bankruptcy of any one partner
- any partner can choose to end the partnership immediately without notice to the other partners, unless remaining partners elect to continue
- all partners must have free access to the bank account and are entitled to take part in managing the business
- partnership decisions may be made by a majority of the partners, except that all partners must consent to a new partner being admitted as well as any change in the nature of the business
- no partner can be expelled from the partnership
- partners must not compete with the partnership; if they engage in any business on their own account in the same broad field of activity as the partnership, any income from this must be paid to the partnership
- all partners are regarded as 'agents' of the partnership and can take decisions and enter into commitments to which the partnership is bound

---

The need for a written agreement

A partnership in any field can be plagued by problems, and general practice is no exception. Although a written agreement offers no panacea, it at least lays down ground rules which can help to resolve, if not avoid, problems. Once these rules are established, it is only sensible to take a step further by writing them down clearly and unambiguously so that all partners know exactly where they stand.

Partnership disputes are widespread and can present particularly intractable problems. GP partnerships typically experience enough problems and difficulties in normal times. The continual changes in regulations and employment law and the resultant paperwork have increased these problems and placed further pressures on GP partnerships. Whilst an agreement cannot prevent disputes, it can help to avoid many common problems and frequently resolve those which occur by specifying procedures to be followed when a dispute arises or a partnership breaks up.

A written agreement should not slavishly follow some prescribed standard format, but it must reflect the explicit wishes of the partners; only they know how they want to work together, the practice's circumstances and what problems need to be addressed.

What should be included in a written agreement

No written agreement, no matter how comprehensive can be expected to define all the rights and obligations of the partners; many of these have to be inferred from their day-to-day working relations. Nevertheless, there is a well-established framework that is widely used and this normally includes the clauses covered by the headings in Box 5.2 opposite. Strictly speaking many standard clauses covered by these headings are not necessary because the rights or obligations they assign are either prescribed by the Partnership Act 1890 or are always implied – for example, the obligation to be just and faithful in all dealings with one's partners, and to act in good faith towards each other (*see* Box 5.3). Nevertheless it is probably advisable to include them in the agreement.

A written and comprehensive partnership agreement should ensure equity for all partners and reasonable security. Equity does not necessarily imply equality; an equitable partnership agreement should ensure that all partners are treated fairly. For example, the list sizes of individual partners should have no significance in respect of each partner's rights and obligations. It is taken as evidence of good faith if a new partner is able to acquire a comparable list size as soon as reasonably practicable.

The notes below outline issues that need to be addressed and what should be covered under each heading.

Date, name, title and address

Any agreement should specify a date of commencement which may be earlier than the current date if it reflects an existing partnership, or a later

---

Box 5.2: Main headings in a partnership agreement

- date of document
- name, title and address of the partnership
- date when partnership commenced
- nature of the practice's business
- duration of partnership
- practice premises
- partnership capital
- partnership expenses
- partnership income
- sharing the profits
- attending to the affairs of the practice
- managing practice staff
- partnership decisions
- partnership taxation
- holidays and study leave
- maternity provisions
- prolonged incapacity and sickness
- voluntary and compulsory retirement from the partnership
- restrictive covenants
- defence body membership
- banking arrangements
- accounts
- arbitration/conciliation

---

date if it relates to a new partnership. It must be signed by all partners before it is dated; any liability will begin on the commencement date, not the date of agreement, unless both are the same.

The agreement should also include the name under which the partnership will practice, and the addresses of the surgery premises. If the partnership uses any name which does not consist of the true surnames of all partners, the true names of each partner must be included on letter headings, invoices, etc. and displayed in each surgery, to meet the requirements of the Business Names Act 1985.

Box 5.3: A breach of good faith

A new partner joins a practice with a satisfactory partnership agreement. After two or three months, he suggests to the senior partner that it would be a good idea to employ a further practice nurse, adding that he knows someone who would be suitable. The senior partner agrees, and the practice nurse is taken on. The nurse becomes pregnant, and it is revealed subsequently that she is the live-in girlfriend of the new partner. According to the senior partner, a lot of patients are outraged by the situation, and he insists that the nurse stops work and, in fact, wants to dismiss her. According to the partnership agreement, no member of staff can be dismissed without the agreement of all the partners, and therefore the nurse remains on the payroll until such time as she goes on maternity leave. On the basis of advice from the partnership's solicitors, the other partners override the junior partner's opposition on the grounds that his original action, in recommending his girlfriend as an employee without disclosing his relationship with her, was in breach of the obligation to act in good faith towards his partners.

From the BMA's files ...

The nature of the business

A possible wording for this clause is that the partners 'will carry on the profession of NHS general medical practice'. It is essential to specify the nature of the business because this limits the extent to which each partner is liable as an agent of the firm. Otherwise, the liabilities arising from some other quite separate and extraneous business activity undertaken by one partner might be incurred by the other partners, even though they had no direct interest or involvement in this other business. Box 5.4 illustrates the kind of problem that can arise.

Duration of partnership

There is no advantage in limiting duration; doing so reduces the security of all partners and can encourage them to compete among themselves in anticipation of the agreements termination. Thus a partnership should be

---

Box 5.4: Extent of a partnership's liabilities: a partner's wider interests

A GP of 15 years standing, who had worked solely in a three-man practice, started a business outside the practice with which the other two partners had no dealings, financial or otherwise. In 1991, two years after the business started, it went into receivership ...

The GP's assets were liquidated to satisfy his personal debts, and these included his share in the partnership business, its equipment, premises, etc.

From the BMA's files ...

Box 5.5: Duration of partnership

The Partnership Acts 1890 states that every partnership is dissolved in respect of all partners by the death or bankruptcy of any partner, unless there is agreement to the contrary. This is why every partnership agreement covering more than two partners should include a provision to the contrary.

'The partnership shall continue during the joint lives of the partners. The death, retirement, expulsion or bankruptcy of any partner shall not determine the partnership as regards the other partners'.

---

of indefinite duration: for the joint lives of all partners, or any two or more of them (*see* Box 5.5). Failure to state the duration of a partnership will render it a partnership at will which will mean that it can be dissolved at any time at the choice of any partner. However, once a partnership is created, it can be dissolved at any time by *mutual* consent.

Practice premises

An incoming partner should clarify ownership of surgery premises and any prospective liability to purchase a share. If the existing partners have a large investment in property and are seeking a contribution from

---

Box 5.6: Valuing the premises

A practice agreement should specify the basis on which the premises will be valued if a partner dies or resigns. Whatever basis is used, the agreement should state that goodwill must be excluded from the valuation.

---

a new partner, then he or she should seek *independent legal and financial advice*.

A new partner who is buying an equal share of the premises is entitled to an equal share of HA or Health Board direct reimbursement under the rent and rates scheme, even though parity in profit share may not be reached for several years. This important matter is often neglected if a practice simply treats this reimbursement as income and pays it into the partnership account before calculating profit shares.

The agreement should specify which partners are 'property owners'. If there is a lease or licence arrangement between the property-owning partners and other partners, it should be made only on the basis of legal advice and it is preferable that these arrangements are evidenced in a separate legal document. It is preferable that the partnership agreement defines the owners and confirms the rights of the others to use the practice premises, and that the remaining partners should have a continuing right to use the premises for, say, three months if the property owner(s) leave the partnership.

Rent and rates payments from the Health Authority or Health Board should normally be paid into the partnership's bank account, being the property of the partnership as a whole (*see* Chapter 6 for a description of alternative ways of distributing these payments among partners, depending upon their shares in ownership of the property).

Partnership capital

This normally includes all property, equipment, drugs, surgery fittings and furniture, together with any cash used as working capital. An incoming partner will buy a share of these assets and also contribute to the practice's working capital. Partners normally own shares of the assets (apart from the premises) in the same proportion as their share in the profits. The written agreement should specify how shares in the partnership's capital are divided among the partners (*see* Box 5.7), what constitutes the capital, and also confirm the arrangements for expanding the capital.

Box 5.7: Acrimony over who owned what

Dr A fell out with his partners Drs B and C, and as a consequence, dissolution of the partnership was discussed. There had been considerable discontent between the partners which arose from a long period of study leave taken by Dr A. The partnership did not have a written agreement. When discussions took place about the partnership break-up, it was extremely difficult to disentangle the capital of the partnership from items individually owned by the partners. This sadly led to the demeaning scene of Dr A arguing in front of patients with Drs B and C over who owned which items of surgery equipment and furniture.

There was no statement of the capital assets and no inventory which the three partners could use in their discussions about dissolution. Consequently, the process was accompanied by considerable acrimony.

From the BMA's files ...

Partnership expenses

The agreement should specify which expenses should be paid by the partnership as a whole; typically these should include the cost of practice staff, accounting and banking services, telephone and stationery, and also the costs of occupying and running the premises (rent, rates, heating, lighting, cleaning and maintenance). All these shared expenses should be met before profits are calculated and distributed, and partners should contribute to them in proportion to their profit shares.

Other expenses, such as the costs of the partners' cars and house telephones, are normally paid by individual partners because this arrangement is usually fairer. Whichever arrangement prevails, it should be specified clearly in the agreement so that there can be no ambiguity and uncertainty about this crucial matter.

Partnership income

It is generally held to be advisable to include all earnings from professional practice in the partnership's income, otherwise individual partners might be encouraged to concentrate on those activities rewarded by personal rather than practice income and even compete among themselves for this type of work. However, it is possible with care to arrange a partnership's affairs to enable partners to retain their non-general medical services professional income and not to put the harmony of the partnership at risk.

Certain earnings are normally retained personally because they should not put at risk the collective efforts of the partnership (e.g. the seniority and postgraduate education allowances). Whatever arrangement is agreed, it must be equitable and should be defined in the partnership agreement (*see* Box 5.8).

Box 5.8: 'A postgraduate experience'

A new partner unwittingly signed a partnership agreement which allowed the other two partners to retain their seniority allowances and PGEAs, but required her PGEA to be paid into the 'pool' for distribution among all partners.

From the BMA's files ...

Dividing the profits

Stated simply, the profit (or loss) is the difference between practice income and expenses. The agreement should specify the size of each partner's share of the profits, and how it is calculated and paid. If changes in the share ratios are planned (e.g. a move to parity for a new partner), these need to be stated, including when they should take effect.

Under NHS regulations, for the Health Authority or Health Board to recognize GPs as partners, it must be satisfied that they discharge the duties and exercise the powers of a principal in the partnership and that, unless an approved job sharer, they are entitled to a share of the profits (*see* Box 5.9) based on one of these options:

- if contracted to be available for at least 26 hours a week – a share of not less than one third of the partner with greatest share
- if contracted to be available for between 19 and 26 hours – not less than one quarter of greatest share
- if contracted to be available for between 13 and 19 hours – not less than one fifth of greatest share.

If any partner's share is grossly out of line with his or her contribution to the work of the practice, a concealed sale of goodwill may be deemed to have taken place (*see* Box 5.10).

Box 5.9: Salaried partners

This description is a contradiction in terms as far as it applies to any independent contractor. Someone is either a partner with all the rights and obligations which this entails, or they are not, in which case they are not a principal and the practice is not entitled, for example, to be paid a BPA (and its related allowances) for that doctor.

Box 5.10: Sale of goodwill is prohibited

The Medical Practices Committee (MPC) is responsible for issues concerning the sale of goodwill. Since 1948 GPs have been forbidden to sell the 'goodwill' of an NHS practice, 'goodwill' being the established custom of popularity of a practice. Examples of deemed sales of goodwill include:

- the premises are sold for substantially more than might have been expected if they had not previously been used for general practice
- a significant payment is made other than for undertaking partnership duties
- a partner receives a significantly less amount for his or her services than might reasonably be expected.

In particular, the MPC looks to see if the balance between profit share and workload is equitable.

The MPC may regard the following as evidence of a sale of goodwill:

- a new partner does not reach parity in the partnership profits within three years
- one or more partners is permitted to do less than a fair share of the practice workload
- one or more partners get longer or shorter holidays, or exceptionally is or is not entitled to study leave
- if, after a reasonable assessment period, a partner is restricted in taking onto his or her list any patient who chooses to register with him or her
- if the terms of expulsion, retirement or dissolution are not mutual.

Any GP about to join a practice who is concerned about a possible sale of goodwill may submit the terms of the proposed partnership to the Medical Practices Committee.

An incoming partner's share should be sufficient for it to be more than he or she might have earned as an assistant: this share should increase each year so that parity is reached within a reasonable time span, normally three years. He or she should not be prevented from taking a fair share of new patients onto his or her list (*see* Box 5.11).

Attending to the affairs of the practice

The agreement should state the time and attention which partners are expected to give to the work of the partnership, especially if one partner is allowed to give less time than others to it. If the partners are required to devote their whole time to the practice, it is advisable for the agreement to stipulate that they should not engage in any other business or accept any office (e.g. local councillor) without the consent of the other partners.

In the present climate, time spent on medical politics (e.g. as an LMC member or as a GMSC member) should be allowed for in the agreement, preferably before the issue has to be faced.

Managing practice staff

The agreement should specify who carries responsibility for staff matters. It is advisable that staff employed by the partnership should be engaged and dismissed only with the consent of all partners, otherwise a dismissed employee could pursue a successful dismissal claim against the partnership as a whole if all partners have not agreed on the dismissal (*see* Box 5.13). It is also essential that the agreement should prevent one partner answering or sending letters concerning employment matters without the consent of the other partners. In any circumstances, hastily written and ill considered letters often cause problems.

Partnership decisions

According to the Partnership Act 1890 differences of opinion in the partnership are settled by majority decision unless the agreement specifies some other arrangement. A partnership must decide whether decisions are to be taken on the basis of majority voting and, if so, what size majority is required to endorse different types of decision.

Box 5.11: Exploiting a junior partner

Extract from a Health Authority General Manager's letter:

"Dear Dr C
In reply to your request for information on the practice's arrangements for allocating patients to each partner's list, I can confirm that patients are divided:

Patients with surname	To doctor
A – end of Lane	A
Le – end of Watson	B
all remaining patients	C

I hope this information is helpful"

From the BMA's files ...

Box 5.12: Discrimination is prohibited

It is unlawful for a partnership of any size to discriminate on the grounds of sex or marital status, and for a partnership of six or more partners to discriminate on grounds of colour, race, nationality (including citizenship) or ethnic or national origins:

* when appointing a new partner
* in the terms on which the new partner is offered a partnership
* by refusing, or deliberately neglecting, to offer a partnership

and where someone is already a partner:

* in the way he or she is afforded access to any benefits, facilities or services; or by refusing, or deliberately neglecting, to afford access to those benefits, facilities and services; or
* by dismissing the partner, or treating him or her unfavourably in any other way.

Box 5.13: Staff dismissal led to partnership rift

A busy urban four-doctor partnership decided to make several significant changes in the organization of its practice staff. These included introducing a new computer system, leading to an enlarged job description for the practice manager.

The senior receptionist was not happy about the changes and felt that the practice manager was usurping some of her work. Tension grew and came to a head when she had a blazing row with one of the partners. The latter discussed it with the other partner on duty and dismissed the receptionist that day. When the other two partners were informed, they felt the decision had been too hasty.

The senior receptionist immediately applied to the industrial tribunal claiming unfair dismissal. Strains appeared within the partnership and it split into two before the hearing. The two partners who had not been involved in the dismissal believed they had no responsibility or financial liability with regard to the industrial tribunal case.

The tribunal found in favour of the dismissed receptionist who was awarded almost £10 000. The doctors who had not been responsible for the dismissal believed that they were not liable for the payment. But lack of any reference in the partnership agreement to the dismissal of staff, meant that all four partners were jointly responsible and liable to contribute to the damages.

From the BMA's files ...

How this question is approached usually depends on partnership size. In a partnership of three, partners may opt for unanimity on all decisions, whereas a partnership of six may consider the unanimity is too difficult to achieve and may regard a majority of four to two as a satisfactory basis for decisions. Whatever approach is adopted should be specified in the agreement. Where there are job-share partners, the agreement should specify whether they exercise a half or whole vote each.

Irrespective of how a partnership approaches routine decision making, major decisions which affect key features of the agreement should be taken only if there is unanimity. The nature (i.e. what subjects they relate to) of such decisions should be defined in the agreement.

Taxation

Prior to 1996/97 liability for the income tax on the whole of the practice's net profits was a joint and several liability for each partner. Tax and NI for staff wages are however still a joint and several liability for each partner. The partnership agreement should therefore provide for enough funds to be set aside for tax liabilities, preferably in a separate bank or building society account designated for this purpose.

Box 5.14: Joint and several liability

Dr C, Dr D and Dr E were in a dispensing partnership. Dr E ran the dispensing part of the practice and Drs C and D did not question his figures or returns for this. Subsequently Drs C and D were horrified to find that Dr E had been fraudulent to the tune of over £500 000. Dr E did not account to Drs C and D for this money. The Health Authority did however request repayment and the Inland Revenue demanded tax on it and Drs C and D were held jointly and severally liable for repayment.

Holiday and study leave

Each partner's eligibility for leave should be on an equitable basis (*see* Box 5.15). When a locum is employed to cover holiday or study leave, expenses should normally be met by the partnership as a whole. It is advisable for the agreement to restrict the number of partners who can be on leave concurrently and the maximum length of unbroken leave which can be taken.

Sickness and pregnancy

Partnerships can make various arrangements to pay for locums employed during prolonged absences. A simple method is for the absent partner to pay all the locum expenses. However, it is increasingly common for the partnership as a whole to pay the first few weeks of these expenses.

> **Box 5.15: Surprised by holiday arrangements**
>
> In a three-partner practice, a new partner signed a partnership agreement whereby he agreed to cover holiday periods etc. The three partners also agreed that they would cover each other's holidays to avoid the cost of hiring locums. Unfortunately for the new partner he had neglected to take account of the fact that the other two partners were married to each other and took their holidays together. As a result the new partner found himself providing continuous cover for the whole practice for at least six weeks each year.
>
> **From the BMA's files ...**

A partnership will infringe the Sex Discrimination Act if a pregnant partner is treated less favourably than a male partner with a distinctly male incapacity. Therefore a partner on maternity leave should not have to meet the full cost of a locum unless this arrangement also applies to sick leave. Box 5.16 outlines the BMA's recommended maternity leave arrangements.

Additional payments made by the Health Authority or Health Board during sickness or confinement should be paid to the absent partner if he or she is responsible for locum expenses.

The question of how long the partnership or the individual partner pays locum expenses needs to be decided in relation to the arrangements for insurance cover for income protection and/or locum expenses.

Leaving the partnership

The agreement should specify the conditions under which partners may retire, including the required period of notice. It is usually simpler if the period of notice expires on a quarter-day so as to coincide with quarterly Health Authority or Health Board payments. Ideally, a retiring partner should be allowed some discretion in selecting a date for retirement which is most favourable for tax purposes. The notice itself should not be less than three months because Health Authorities and Health Boards are entitled to three months' notice before removing a GP's name from the NHS medical list.

According to the 1890 Partnership Act, a partner cannot be expelled by a majority decision unless the agreement permits this to happen. Thus the

---

Box 5.16: Recommended maternity leave arrangements

- 14 weeks absence should be regarded as a minimum entitlement and the pregnant partner should have the right to determine for herself when the period of absence should start, in consultation with her own GP

- the practice should consider the question of funding the cost of a locum to cover the actual workload of the pregnant partner not merely her hours of availability

- the partnership should agree on a maximum period of absence following which the partner's failure to return to work may justify compulsory expulsion from the partnership

- the exercise of a partner's right to maternity leave should not abolish her entitlement to *pro rata* holiday and sickness leave

- adoption: the partnership agreement should specify leave arrangements

A partnership agreement which provides for maternity leave on terms which are less advantageous than sick leave could be construed as evidence of indirect sex discrimination.

---

agreement should contain a clause which makes provision for the expulsion of a partner in specific circumstances such as prolonged incapacity, mental ill-health, removal or suspension from the medical register or NHS medical list, gross breaches of the agreement and bankruptcy. Although such a clause would confer a right to expel a partner in certain specific circumstances, like any clause it may be waived by mutual consent.

Most agreements require a partner to retire after a period of prolonged incapacity which prevents him or her from doing a fair share of the work for a period of six to 12 months. Naturally most partnerships wish to be as generous as possible in such circumstances, but because prolonged absence imposes a considerable burden on colleagues, it may be advisable to require an incoming partner to produce evidence of good health before the partnership agreement is signed. Any sickness provision should be seen to be reasonable and preferably have provision for independent medical opinion.

Retirement

All GPs are required to retire from NHS practice by or on their 70th birthday. Thus it is sensible to include in the agreement a requirement that each partner retire from the practice by or on this compulsory retirement date. It may be advisable also to include a clause which allows a partner to continue to practice as a partner in a non-NHS capacity beyond a certain age, if other partners agree.

The partnership should agree on a clear and fair policy on retirement before individual problems arise; difficulties can occur if a practice only considers the issue of its retirement policy when the retirement of an individual partner is under discussion.

The issue of retirement can be particularly contentious for any partnership. Younger and older partners often express differing views on the subject, and a partner's perception of the issue may alter as retirement approaches. Young doctors entering a partnership often prefer a clause requiring compulsory retirement at a specific age such as 60 years, because it reduces the risk of them having to support an old and ailing partner who is increasingly unable to do a fair share of the work. Such a clause may be attractive to partners when they themselves are comparatively young, but it becomes less attractive as retirement approaches.

Restrictive covenants

NHS legislation prohibits the purchase or sale of goodwill, but did not abolish goodwill as such. Thus it is legal to protect goodwill by reasonable restrictions on the future activities of a departing partner. Such restrictions are commonplace and usually enforceable. But any restraint must be entirely reasonable.

Any restrictive covenant must apply equally to all partners and relate only to work normally undertaken by a GP, and its duration should not be too long. Any restriction from working in a defined area must be reasonable; there should be a significant number of patients near to the boundary and it should not include any large concentrations of population which are of little or no significance to the practice. It may be advisable for the agreement to refer to the practice area map which would normally be a reasonable area in which to restrict an outgoing partner from practising. The map itself could be included in the agreement.

It is preferable to have a limited restraint clause which is capable of being enforced rather than a more Draconian one which is unenforcable. Moreover, it is important to note that, in recent years, courts have taken an increasingly critical view of restrictive covenants.

The MPC has issued important advice on restraint clauses (*see* Box 5.17 below), particularly in relation to the length of time and distance specified.

Box 5.17: Restrictive covenants: advice from the MPC

- the MPC looks at restrictive covenants to see if they are reasonable and mutual in their application. If the provisions are regarded as unreasonable or too restrictive the MPC may consider this to be evidence of a sale of goodwill

- the MPC, in forming its opinion, normally regards as an acceptable upper limit a restrictive covenant which prevents a doctor engaging in NHS general practice and/or treating certain patients within a radius of two miles from the main premises for a period of two years. But variations may be justified by special circumstances

- the MPC would also consider there may be evidence of sale of goodwill if the radius and period were both reasonable but there was some extra restriction on a doctor acting within it in any capacity other than a GP; for example, if it prevented the doctor from filling a hospital appointment within the radius

---

Defence body subscriptions

Each partner must be required to be a member of a medical defence organization, or hold appropriate medical indemnity insurance whilst a partner.

Banking arrangements

The agreement should name the partnership's bankers and specify the arrangements for signing cheques. All partners should be signatories to the account. The agreement should provide however for at least two signatories for cheques over a set amount.

Box 5.18 shows a not untypical inequitable agreement in respect of a partnership's banking arrangement.

Box 5.18: Extract from a partnership agreement signed in 1990

'The partnership bank account shall be under the sole control of the principal partner and any cheque thereon shall be signed by him alone and the junior partner hereby appoints the principal partner as his attorney for all purposes in connection with the operation of the said bank account and the signing of cheques drawn thereon'

From the BMA's files ...

Partnership accounts

The agreement should name the partnership's accountants and specify arrangements for drawing up the accounts, including the date of the practice's financial year. It is normal to require all partners to sign the annual accounts for them to be binding.

All partners must have free access to the partnership's accounts and records. Any denial of access to any partner is strong *prima facie* evidence that the doctor concerned is in fact an employee, not a partner. It may be advisable to include in the agreement a provision that all partners and their agents (e.g. personal accountants) should have copies of the accounts.

Arbitration

However carefully drafted, no agreement can cover all contingencies. Disputes and differences of opinion can occur even in the most harmonious partnership. Most should be resolved within the partnership, sometimes with advice or assistance from the local BMA office, or even with assistance from an independent conciliator. Traditionally, the BMA has advised doctors to make provision in their partnership agreements for disputes to be referred by mutual agreement to independent arbitration. In practice the use of arbitration should be very rare indeed. It is almost invariably an expensive process (usually much more costly than initially anticipated), more legalistic than is often assumed, and, perhaps more important, often accompanies a final breakdown in the partnership and therefore does not contribute to its continuation (*see* Box 5.19). Thus, though arbitration may be appropriate in certain specific circumstances, these are more limited that is generally assumed.

The best advice to follow is for all partners to consider carefully the possible consequences of any action they may be contemplating, individually or collectively, which may precipitate arbitration and lead ultimately to the dissolution of the partnership. Any type of legal action, including arbitration, is almost invariably a costly option and is often associated with the break up of the partnership.

Box 5.19: Sledgehammer to crack a nut?

In a partnership of seven, a majority of partners (six to one) decided to purchase pregnancy-testing equipment to the value of £250. The one partner opposed was very unhappy with the decision. He deemed this expenditure to be unnecessary and inappropriate, believing the provision of a pregnancy-testing service would result in its use prior to abortion. He also objected to the provision of such a service free of charge. He could not prevent his partners from offering this service to their patients, but he did not see why they should be doing so at the expense of the partnership; that is, partly at his own expense. The matter was referred to arbitration. The arbitration decision was lengthy and costly, and led ultimately to the dissolution of the partnership. All parties incurred several thousands of pounds of legal costs and the only outcome was a dissolution which was also costly.

From the BMA's files ...

6   Surgery Premises

NHS general practice differs from other professions in that a substantial proportion of the cost of providing premises is directly met from public funds. This is because successive governments have wished to ensure high standard surgery premises are generally available. Of course, NHS GPs also work within a different financial framework to those of other professions. They cannot simply raise income to fund premises by increasing their charges to clients, unlike for example accountants or solicitors. However, because public funds are at stake, the reimbursement of GPs' premises costs is subject to detailed and stringent controls, including rules specifying the amount of space eligible for reimbursement and how an appropriate level of rent reimbursement is assessed by the district valuer. In practice, no single element in the reimbursement scheme is free from public scrutiny or control. Box 6.1 summarizes these controls.

> **Box 6.1: Health Authority and Health Board controls over use of public funds for surgery premises**
>
> - government's district valuer advises on valuations to assess level of notional rent
> - government's district valuer advises on valuations relating to cost rent scheme
> - Red Book specifies minimum standards and maximum size of surgery premises eligible for reimbursement
> - 'prescribed percentage' set by the Health Department determines level of cost rent payments

GPs' terms of service require them to provide adequate surgery accommodation 'having regard to the circumstances' of the practice and to allow this to be inspected by the Health Authority or Health Board and/or LMC. Virtually every GP is eligible to be reimbursed rent and rates for their surgery premises. But the Health Authority or Health Board has to be satisfied that the use of existing premises, their enlargement or a move to new premises, is in the interests of the NHS.

Although GPs can expect a high proportion of premises' costs to be directly refunded by the Health Authority or Health Board, they often meet some of these costs themselves.

Surgery premises are usually provided in one of these ways:

- rented from a private landlord
- rented from a local authority
- rented from a health authority (often referred to as health centres)
- owner-occupied by an individual GP or partners
- newly developed under the 'cost rent' scheme and owner-occupied by an individual GP or partners, or rented from a third party.

Rented surgeries

GPs who rent a surgery from a landlord can recover the cost of the rent from the Health Authority or Health Board. An appropriate rent, as assessed by the district valuer, is repaid in full. If the premises are not used wholly for NHS work (e.g. if a part is sublet), an equivalent proportion of the rent is not reimbursed.

Health centres

The rent of GPs practising from health centres owned by health authorities (together with their business and water rates) is normally paid by the Health Authority or Health Board directly to the authority. Because it is not paid out from the practice's own funds and subsequently reimbursed, GPs should take particular care to ensure that both the rent and the equivalent amount of direct reimbursement are shown in their accounts. (Otherwise, if their accounts should be selected by the Inland Revenue for its anonymized sample of tax returns, their actual expenses will be assessed wrongly and this will adversely affect the Review Body's estimate of the level of average expenses due to be repaid indirectly to the profession as a whole.) The practice accountant should understand why these payments and reimbursements must be shown correctly.

Owner-occupied surgeries

In many cases, surgeries will not be rented from a third party but owned instead by the GPs themselves, either individually or in partnership. A rent allowance (notional rent) is therefore paid to recompense them for the use of their privately-owned surgery for NHS purposes.

Valuation of GP premises

At present, incoming partners buying a share of practice premises must only make a contribution based upon the *vacant possession* valuation of a building. Otherwise a sale of goodwill might be deemed to arise. Given current reduced property values, such a valuation may not represent the full investment made in premises by an outgoing partner. Thus a conflict of interests can occur over valuations between incoming and outgoing partners.

Notional rent allowance

Notional rent is paid on owner-occupied surgeries that are neither new nor developed within the scope of the cost rent scheme; it is based on a district valuer's assessment of the current market rent which may reasonably be expected to be paid for the premises. It is paid quarterly or monthly to the practice and is reviewed triennially. Until the recent decline in property values, this triennial review normally led to an increased notional rent and many practices became accustomed over many years to a steady increase in its level. Any practice which is not satisfied with its notional rent assessment may appeal against it.

Other reimbursements for premises

Health Authorities reimburse other costs relating to surgery premises, as shown in Box 6.2.

Box 6.2: Rent and rates scheme: types of direct reimbursement

- cost rents
- notional rents
- uniform business rates
- water rates
- sewerage rates
- sewerage charges
- water meter installation costs and charges
- refuse collection charges

These payments should be regularly and correctly claimed; practices are known to have foregone many thousands of pounds of income because they have failed to submit claims.

Some Health Authorities have introduced arrangements for paying rates and similar charges directly, which can improve a practice's cash flow. However, these payments and reimbursements, although they appear to be 'notional', must not be 'netted out' and thereby omitted from the practice's accounts.

Partnerships

It is usual for partnerships to own the surgery premises. But it is not uncommon for the partners to own them in differently sized proportions to the ratios which define their profit shares. For example, in a six-doctor partnership, two may be part-time or partially retired GPs not involved in surgery ownership, leaving the other four partners owning the building. One way of clarifying and simplifying ownership arrangements is to make a clear separation between the partnership formed for the purposes of providing general medical services, and that formed to own and run the premises. The 'clinical' partnership can then treat the ownership of the premises as a quite separate exercise from the profit sharing activities of the partnership. The 'property owning' partnership charges rent to the profit sharing partnership, which in turn receives notional rent income from the Health Authority or Health Board. Alternatively, notional rent may be received by only the property owning partners.

Improvement grants

Grants are available for improving surgeries and these are subject to Health Authority or Health Board cash limits in the same way as cost rent schemes and practice staff reimbursement. These grants are paid only if a Health Authority or Health Board has given prior approval to an improvement scheme and if the same expenditure is not also claimed as allowable expenditure against income tax. GPs should obtain advice from their practice accountant on whether to opt for an improvement grant or a tax allowance. If part of the cost of an improvement project does not qualify for a grant, tax relief can be claimed on the residual amount.

Taxation

The notional rent allowance is paid to GPs whose privately owned surgeries are used for NHS general practice. It is essential for tax purposes that this is not treated or regarded as 'rent' in the usual sense of the word. In particular, it should not be treated as the private unearned income of GPs and it should not be included in the property section of the tax return. Otherwise, it could have a detrimental effect on how it is taxed and on whether retirement relief is granted for capital gains purposes.

New surgery development: the cost rent scheme

Most new or 'substantially improved' surgeries are funded by the cost rent scheme. Instead of being reimbursed at the current market rate (known as 'notional rent'), a GP may be reimbursed the cost of providing separate purpose-built premises (known as 'cost rent') if they are:

- completely new
- acquired and substantially modified
- already used and substantially modified.

An essential feature of the cost rent scheme is its recognition of the difference between the cost of providing an existing surgery and that of an entirely new or substantially improved surgery. It does not directly reimburse the actual interest paid on a loan for the cost of a building project. A practice should therefore ensure that its project is financially sound before entering into any commitment. It should be certain that the cost of servicing and repaying the loan can be met from the cost rent income, other practice income or (if necessary) funds from private sources.

The cost rent allowance is calculated by multiplying the cost of the project by a 'prescribed' percentage: for either a variable or fixed rate loan, according to the particular funding arrangement employed. To illustrate, if a project's total cost is £800 000 and the current fixed rate for the purpose of calculating cost rent is eight per cent, the annual cost rent payment to the practice is £64 000.

The four main cost components of a cost rent project are:

- buying the land
- erecting or modifying the building
- architectural and other professional fees
- bridging loan interest.

Because Health Authority and Health Board funds for cost rent projects are cash limited, before entering into any commitments practices should:

- obtain Health Authority/Health Board agreement 'in principle' to the project
- ascertain its priority in the Health Authority/Health Board overall programme
- find out when cost rent payments will actually be made.

Not only must approval be obtained for the project, but the Health Authority or Health Board should state whether it has sufficient funds for the scheme within its development programme and when they will be available.

The Health Authority's or Health Board's formal written offer should:

- confirm that the project is accepted for cost rent reimbursement
- specify the method used to calculate the level of reimbursement
- give an interim estimate of the level of reimbursement (interim cost rent)
- give a target date when reimbursement should start.

This written offer will be conditional upon the project being completed within a given timescale; if this is not possible the Health Authority or Health Board may withdraw approval (without any obligation to meet any expenses the practice has already incurred).

GPs must ensure that they have planning permission and that their architects are aware of the cost rent scheme, particularly its limits on size and building costs as set out in the Red Book. These cost limits are defined for each Health Authority or Health Board and reflect regional variations in building costs.

Cost rent limits

The maximum amount that can be spent on building a surgery is strictly limited. Many practices find it difficult to keep within these limits and have had to finance significant shortfalls from their own resources.

When the Health Authority or Health Board has determined the total costs that can be included in the scheme, it calculates the amount of cost rent to be reimbursed by multiplying that sum by a 'prescribed percentage'. There are two percentage rates 'prescribed' by the Health Department: a variable rate which is reviewed annually and a fixed rate which is reviewed quarterly.

The variable rate of reimbursement applies to projects funded by a variable rate loan, whereas the fixed rate applies to those wholly or mainly funded from a practice's own money or a fixed rate loan. If the fixed rate loan includes an option to switch to a variable rate, the fixed rate of reimbursement prevails until this choice is made.

Raising money for a cost rent project

When the project has been approved by the Health Authority or Health Board, the next step is to raise money to fund it. Cost rent payments to a practice are calculated according to a fixed formula (which may be subject to some minor modifications) that takes no account of how the practice raises its funds. The actual process of obtaining the loan, and agreeing interest and repayment rates is a totally separate matter. This distinction is crucial. The 'prescribed' percentage rate is deemed by the Health Department to be a reasonable average level of return on capital; it takes no account of the idiosyncrasies of the loan market or the varying ability of practices to raise loans. Thus there may be a significant difference between the income received from the cost rent allowance and the expenditure incurred on the loan.

Banks, insurance companies and building societies provide long-term loans for cost rent projects. Although the mortgage offers security to the lender in the event of a practice defaulting on its loan, it could be argued that the actual 'security' is the income paid to the practice through the cost rent scheme. Normally this income will continue to be paid uninterrupted for as long as a surgery is deemed by the Health Authority or Health Board as being used to provide NHS practice, unless the practice opts to change to notional rent. Nevertheless, the lender will wish to be satisfied that the practice can service and repay the loan according to its agreed terms, because the cost rent income can be less than the cost of servicing the debt. If there is a shortfall between cost rent income and loan repayment, this has to be met from practice income unless the partners have access to private resources. This current or future liability must be assessed at the outset by the partners according to their personal circumstances so that each partner can decide how the shortfall should be funded.

Changing to notional rent

The Red Book recognizes that current market rent (notional rent) is unlikely to produce initially a higher level of reimbursement than cost rent, therefore cost rent is paid until a practice opts to change to notional rent. But once this switch is made it cannot be reversed.

A review of notional rent can be requested:

• every three years from the operative date of the cost rent if the premises are owned by the practice

OR

• (if the premises are leased by the practice) when the rent due under the lease is reviewed or a new lease is entered into at the expiry of the existing lease.

Notional rent will be reviewed every three years after the date of assessment.

The decision to switch depends on several factors. Clearly, notional rent must exceed cost rent, and in the longer term a practice may feel relatively secure in the knowledge that property values and rents have (with some notable exceptions) tended to rise steadily year on year. However, recent years have witnessed a substantial decline in property and rental values. The average time taken for 'notional rent' to overtake 'cost rent' used to be in the range of seven to nine years. A significant problem has now arisen for those practices who switched from cost to notional rent three years ago, only to find that on triennial review the notional rent has fallen to a level which is below the original cost rent. There are GPs who are now finding that the value of their equity in the premises has fallen below their original investment and, instead of realizing a gain at retirement, are facing the prospect of having to repay a considerable sum to the partnership to reflect this.

Clearly, a practice should assess carefully at the time of review how much more reimbursement would be paid, likely future movements in interest rates and, the projected economic and political climate during the period prior to the next review of the prescribed variable rate.

7 Employing Practice Staff

As employers, GPs are subject to an extensive range of employment law; during the past 25 years some 16 Acts of Parliament have been implemented establishing over 20 new legal rights for individual employees. Only recently, unfair dismissal and redundancy rights have been extended to include anyone with two years' service irrespective of how many hours a week they work.

This plethora of legislation has been enacted by successive governments to encourage a more formal and equitable approach to industrial relations and personnel matters. Other influences affecting this legislation have included comparisons with international standards (e.g. the Equal Pay Act and Sex Discrimination Act, and recent European legislation on maternity leave) and legislation in other fields such as the Race Relations Act. Although this body of employment law is intended to influence personnel practices in all organizations, the special position of the small employer, whose circumstances and resources differ greatly from those of the large organization, has usually been ignored by legislators. There have been some recent minor concessions to size, but nevertheless the totality of employment law imposes a far greater administrative burden on a small employer.

Box 7.1:

Individual rights	Eligibility (length of service)
To be given a minimum period of notice – based on length of service – of termination of employment	One month
To be given written particulars of terms of employment	Two months
To receive equal pay with a member of the opposite sex doing similar work	None – applies immediately
Not to be discriminated against on the grounds of marriage or sex	Any stage from advertising of job
Not to be discriminated against on the grounds of colour, race, nationality, or ethnic or national origins	Any stage from advertising of job
Not to be unfairly dismissed	Two years*
Not to be dismissed on pregnancy or childbirth grounds	None – applies immediately
To take 14 weeks' maternity leave	None – applies immediately
To return to work up to 29 weeks after week in which childbirth occurs	Two years
To have unpaid time off for public duties	None – applies immediately

continued opposite

Box 7.1: *continued*

Individual rights	Eligibility (length of service)
To have time off – with pay – to seek alternative work or to arrange training if made redundant	Two years*
To receive an itemized pay statement	None – applies immediately
To receive on request a written statement of the reason for dismissal	Two years (immediately and automatically if for pregnancy reasons)
To have paid time off for antenatal care	None – applies immediately

* If dismissal is for certain inadmissible reasons – that is, for reasons of trade union membership or activities, maternity or childbirth, or sex or race discrimination – there is no length of service qualification.

The overriding aim of any employer should be to avoid litigation. This can be achieved by good management practice which means taking a more formal approach to many employment matters, such as preparing written employment contracts. For instance, small businesses often fail to issue written contracts of employment to staff (even though the law requires that this should be done) and rely instead on informal and undocumented understandings, which are often a recipe for disaster.

This chapter summarizes the following key aspects of employment legislation:

• the employment contract: what it should contain and how to change it
• statutory maternity leave and pay
• disciplinary and dismissal procedures
• discrimination.

The employment contract

A contract of employment exists as soon as an employee demonstrates an acceptance of an employer's terms and conditions of employment by starting work. Both employer and employee are then bound by the terms offered and accepted. Often the initial agreement is verbal not written, but within two calendar months of any employee starting work the employer is legally obliged to provide a written statement detailing the main terms of employment, including a note on disciplinary procedures.

This written statement must contain the following information:

- names of parties to the contract
- date employment began and statement about continuity of employment
- job title or brief description of the work
- place of work
- pay, scale or rate of remuneration, intervals between payment
- hours of work
- holiday entitlement and holiday pay
- sick pay and sick leave
- pension arrangements
- notice of termination or length of contract
- grievance, disciplinary and appeals procedures (employers with less than 20 employees are exempt from including information on the disciplinary procedure).

It is also advisable, though not obligatory, to include information on:

- retirement policy
- maternity provisions
- health and safety policy.

It is sensible to prepare and issue a comprehensive contract of employment that covers all these subjects. (Members can obtain a model employment contract from their local BMA office.)

Attention paid to preparing a correct contract of employment should prevent unforeseen and unwanted disputes. The actual process of preparing and agreeing a contract should ensure that the practice is reasonably familiar with its legal responsibilities and obligations, and has not unknowingly acted contrary to these at the outset. Moreover, if any dispute should arise and a practice has to defend its personnel practices and policies, its position is greatly strengthened if it can show that it acted in good faith and took reasonable steps to conform with the law.

The statutory requirement to provide written statements on these matters does not have to be supplemented in any way. Although there is no legal obligation to provide a written contract as such, in practice a written statement of the main particulars of employment (together with a policy statement on health and safety) can be regarded as the basis of a written employment contract. The contract as a whole also includes the job description (whether written or not), and also the many informal and undocumented understandings and working practices which inevitably form an important part of any employment contract. An example of these informal and unwritten practices are the arrangements applying to staff coffee and tea breaks.

A written contract may have to be changed. No difficulties should arise if the correct procedure is adopted and the substantive reason for the change is 'reasonable'. There are various ways of changing a contract and the key underlying principle is that an employee should normally consent to any changes before they can become contractually binding, irrespective of whether this consent is implied or, by express agreement, given in advance of, or at the time of the change.

Obviously, an employer should seek to reach agreement on the proposed changes. If consent is obtained this can be given by express agreement, either orally or preferably in writing. In any case, an employer is required to put in writing the changed terms of the contract if they relate to any of the obligatory subjects listed above. Alternatively, consent may be demonstrated by implied agreement which can normally be assumed if an employee continues to work under the new contractual terms without complaint.

The written contract itself may contain provisions that allow for changes in matters such as pay, place of work, working hours and duties of the job. Nevertheless, even if a contract is drafted broadly, an employer must be prepared to show that the change itself is reasonable and was implemented in a reasonable way.

If consent is not forthcoming, even though the employer has made considerable efforts to agree the change with staff, unilateral implementation requires a reasonable period of notice. Normally, any contractual change imposed by an employer without an employee's consent will be a breach of contract, and if this is a fundamental breach (striking at the heart of the contract), an employee may be entitled to claim compensation for unfair dismissal. But by giving sufficient notice of the change, normally at least as long as that required to terminate the contract, it may be possible to avoid these problems. However, even if this length of notice is given, an employer could still be liable to pay compensation for unfair dismissal or redundancy. The advantage of giving adequate notice of change is that the employee is usually left with little or no time to protest after it is actually introduced.

In summary, the reasonableness of any change to an employment contract is subject to both a procedural test and a substantive test. Two questions have to be addressed and be capable of being answered in the affirmative:

• have you proceeded in a reasonable way by seeking agreement and giving adequate notice?

• is the proposed change itself a reasonable one to make in the particular circumstances of the business?

Statutory maternity rights

Most practices employ only a small number of staff, a large majority of whom are women. The employment rights of the expectant mother are intricate and stringent; thus, any employer can face serious administrative problems if staff become pregnant.

The six main employment rights of the expectant mother are:

• not to be unreasonably refused paid time off work for antenatal care (applicable to all employees irrespective of length of service)

• to take 14 weeks' maternity leave

• to take 40 weeks' maternity leave and return to work if she has at least two years' service

• to receive 18 weeks' statutory maternity pay (SMP) if she has 26 weeks' recent continuous employment and normal weekly earnings above the NI lower limit

• to complain of unfair dismissal if dismissed because of pregnancy or childbirth

• to return to work after absence on account of pregnancy or confinement.

This area of employment law is complex for both employer and employee. It is vital that GPs obtain detailed guidance on how to ensure an employee obtains her statutory maternity rights; each practice should have a copy of the Department of Social Security free booklet *Employer's Manual on Statutory Maternity Pay.* Any mistake, even if due to ignorance or misunderstanding of the law, could lead to a tribunal case and costly compensatory award. Industrial tribunals are assiduous in upholding pregnant employees' rights and impose severe penalties in cases where unfair dismissals have occurred because of pregnancy or childbirth.

Disciplinary procedures and dismissal

Employers are required to include details of their disciplinary procedures, and the rules governing an appeal against disciplinary action, in their employment contracts, or to specify where these are to be found. (Although employers with fewer than 20 employees are exempted from this requirement it is advisable for all of them to do so.)

Disciplinary rules and procedures should promote fairness and order in the treatment of individual employees. They help a practice to run effectively by setting standards of conduct and performance, and ensuring that these are followed; they should not be seen primarily as a means of imposing sanctions. Their main purpose should be to emphasize and encourage improvements in individual employees' conduct and performance.

Employees who have not completed two years' continuous employment, cannot normally complain of unfair dismissal, except if the dismissal is for an inadmissible reason such as pregnancy or childbirth.

The risk of a successful claim of unfair dismissal (which can involve compensation payments of several thousands of pounds) can be largely avoided if the procedure adopted is fair and reasonable, and the reasons for the dismissal are also fair and reasonable. A practice may have to justify its actions in an industrial tribunal so it is wise to keep detailed documentation throughout.

Several key principles relating to retiring age affect an employee's rights to complain of unfair dismissal:

- if normal retiring age is the same for men and women no one may complain of unfair dismissal after that age, whatever it is
- if there is no normal retiring age, anyone under the age of 65 years may complain of unfair dismissal
- if normal retiring age is discriminatory (e.g. 60 years for women and 62 years for men), anyone under 65 years may complain of unfair dismissal.

Normal retiring age is ascertained from the reasonable expectations of employees and may differ from contractual retiring age. It may also vary between posts and grades.

Redundancy

Redundancy is still rare among practice staff but it has become more commonplace as practices have adjusted to the exigencies of the 1990 contract. Regrettably, unfair dismissals on the pretext of redundancy are more common; it is often thought that redundancy offers a more palatable way of getting rid of an unwanted employee.

If a redundancy occurs, important legal obligations fall upon the employer. Employees have a statutory right to receive redundancy payments and paid time off from work to look for another job if they have at least two years' service and work at least eight hours a week. These same qualifying conditions also determine whether the employee has the right to claim unfair dismissal if a redundancy selection has not been made fairly according to objective criteria.

Under employment legislation redundancy is defined as a dismissal caused by an employer's need to reduce the number of staff. Normally an identifiable area of work should have disappeared or been reduced. A dismissal cannot be regarded as a redundancy if the employer immediately engages a direct replacement. But an employee with different skills or in a different location may be engaged (unless the redundant employee could be required under the contract of employment to work at the other location).

Normally any employee of a practice, when it changes hands, automatically becomes an employee of the 'successor' practice on the same terms and conditions of employment. It is as if the employee's contract had originally been made with the new practice; continuity of employment is preserved, as are any rights acquired under the old contract. So when staff are transferred in this way no dismissal has occurred and thus there is no entitlement to a redundancy payment.

An employer must make a statutory lump sum redundancy payment to any employee with at least two years' continuous service, working at least eight hours a week, who is dismissed because of redundancy.

Self-employed people or members of a partnership do not qualify. Employees on fixed term contracts of at least two years' duration which include, with explicit written agreement, a clause waiving entitlement to redundancy payments are also disqualified.

The amount of the lump sum payments depends on how long the employees have been continuously employed, how these years of service relate to particular age bands, and their weekly pay. An employee does not pay tax on statutory redundancy payment and an employer may set it off against tax as a business expense.

As far as possible, objective criteria, precisely defined and capable of being applied in an independent way, should be used when determining who is to be made redundant. This ensures that employees are not unfairly selected for redundancy. Examples of these criteria include length of service, attendance record, experience and capability. They should be applied consistently by any employer irrespective of the size of the business.

Great care must be taken if a practice is considering a redundancy, otherwise it could be faced with a claim for compensation for unfair dismissal. BMA members should contact their local office at the earliest opportunity for expert advice on how to handle this difficult situation. Far too often redundancy has been used as a pretext for dismissing employees who are not in fact redundant. The consequences of using redundancy to dismiss an employee who should otherwise be dismissed on grounds of inefficiency or incapacity, where there is no genuine redundancy, can be very serious indeed. A successful claim for unfair dismissal can require an employer to pay an employee a five figure compensatory award. This compensation cannot be offset against taxation, nor can any part of it be reimbursed by the Health Authority.

Discrimination in employment

GPs rarely experience any difficulties with the race and sex discrimination laws. Of course, avoiding discrimination *per se* is good management practice. It may seem unlikely that a small business with only a small number of employees (most of whom are women) could be affected in any way. But both the Race Relations Act and the Sex Discrimination Act apply to all employers, irrespective of size. Previously the Sex Discrimination Act applied to all employers apart from those with five employees or fewer; the government recently removed this exemption.

There are two areas where legislation requires employers to act (and to be able to show that they have acted) in a manner that is not discriminatory on grounds of:

- sex and marital status
- colour, race, nationality (including citizenship) or ethnic or national origins.

If a practice's recruitment and selection procedures, together with its employment practices, are properly conducted no difficulties should normally arise. Although sex discrimination legislation was primarily intended to improve the employment status and opportunities of women, GPs, whose practice staff are almost exclusively female, should remember that men have equal rights under this legislation.

The scope and structure of both sex and racial discrimination law are similar. Both specify two types of discrimination (direct and indirect) and both require employers to take essentially the same action so as to ensure their employment practices are neither discriminatory in practice nor capable of being interpreted as such.

Direct discrimination occurs when a person treats another person less favourably on grounds of race (or sex, or both) than he or she treats (or would treat) someone else. It is not necessary to show that the person openly expressed an intention to discriminate: it is possible in many instances to infer that the motive was discriminatory in the light of the circumstances of his or her actions.

Indirect discrimination occurs when the treatment may be equal in a formal sense but is discriminatory in its effects on one sex or particular racial group; for example, an unnecessary stipulation that a cleaner should have certain educational qualifications (e.g. 'O' levels or GCSEs) which are not required for the job. When assessing whether an employer has acted in an indirectly discriminatory manner an industrial tribunal is required to consider whether his or her actions, although formally applied in a non-discriminatory manner, have the effect of being discriminatory.

There are three areas where it is unlawful to discriminate on grounds of race or sex when recruiting staff:

• in the arrangements for deciding who should be offered a job
• in relation to the contractual terms offered
• by refusing or deliberately omitting to offer a person employment.

It is also unlawful for employers to discriminate on grounds of sex or race in promotion or training opportunities, and in relation to any other benefits, facilities or services they provide for employees.

The most important matters on which a practice may need to concentrate are its arrangements for selecting and recruiting staff. The more informal its methods, the greater the risk of being accused of discrimination, particularly on grounds of race. An approach based on an informal 'word of mouth' method can easily leave an employer open to a claim (even from someone unknown to the practice who has not actually applied for a vacancy) that the selection procedure is discriminatory.

8 Working in GP and Community Hospitals

Where to obtain advice and assistance

Many GPs are experiencing problems with their part time hospital contracts. BMA local offices can offer expert advice and assistance to members on these matters. The BMA's General Medical Services Committee has prepared a guidance note, which includes a model contract for GPs providing hospital services. The Association of GP Community Hospitals is another source of advice.

Many GPs do some hospital work, usually in a local GP or community hospital. The contracts under which they work are varied and often include informal understandings which reflect long-standing working arrangements. In the past contractual matters have been seriously neglected and GPs have sometimes virtually given their services free of charge to their local community. However, in recent years GPs have expressed increasing disquiet with their contractual arrangements and some practices have sought to improve these; having seen the NHS embrace the market philosophy they themselves are less willing to allow their goodwill be exploited.

It is advisable to exercise great caution in the present NHS climate before taking any steps to change contractual arrangements. Many GPs in these hospital posts have very little security of tenure, particularly if they work only one or two sessions per week. Local NHS management's response to a practice's proposals to improve contractual arrangements may be very different from what is anticipated; in some circumstances management may decide to reduce the level of services in response to a demand for increased pay. In particular, GPs need to know that NHS

Trusts can choose to offer local contracts which differ from nationally negotiated agreements and do not necessarily contain the same safeguards in respect of job security or annual pay reviews.

GPs should obtain expert advice before raising any proposal with local hospital management. Otherwise they could find themselves unwittingly taking a precipitous or irrevocable step which prejudices their long-term position. In NHS Trusts, GPs should also contact the local negotiating committee (LNC) which negotiates with Trust management on behalf of medical staff.

How GPs are paid for hospital work

Clinical assistant grade

Even though the term 'clinical assistant' is not to be found anywhere in the hospital medical staff terms and conditions of service, this grade is nevertheless covered by the appointment procedures specified in paragraph 94 of these and also by NHS General Whitley Council agreements. When working as a clinical assistant, a GP should be responsible to a consultant and carry an overriding commitment to the hospital service rather than general practice. Thus GPs need to make arrangements to cover their practice obligations during those periods when working as clinical assistants.

Since 1988 the maximum number of notional half days for which a clinical assistant may be contracted is five, unless the doctor is an unrestricted GP principal where the maximum is nine.

Box 8.1:

Under paragraph 61 of the hospital terms and conditions of service a notional half day (i.e. session) is defined as three and a half hours, including travelling time.

Clinical assistant posts are normally 12-month fixed-term contracts and renewed annually. Any emergency and on call duties should be spelt out clearly in the contract.

Box 8.2: Key features of the clinical assistant grade

- travel expenses payable under certain conditions
- limited security of tenure
- study leave at employer's discretion
- pay related not to number of beds but to time commitment of job
- employee status
- no independent clinical responsibility
- no incremental pay scale

Hospital practitioner grade

Applicants for posts in this grade must be GP principals with:

- at least two years' full time (or equivalent) hospital experience in a relevant specialty

OR

- a relevant specialist diploma and five years' experience as a clinical assistant

OR

- other equivalent experience.

Box 8.3: Key features of the hospital practitioner grade

- study leave entitlement of 30 days in three years
- emergency and on call duties should be specified in the contract
- hospital terms and conditions of service apply
- travel expenses paid in some circumstances
- security of tenure
- incremental pay scale
- no independent clinical responsibility

Each post has to be advertised and its commitment cannot exceed five sessions per week. The qualifications and experience required of a post-holder depend on both the post and the views of local consultants. Hospital practitioners do not have independent clinical responsibility and are therefore supervised by consultants. Hospital doctors' terms and conditions of service apply.

Staff fund arrangements

A staff fund is based on a local GP or community hospital and is made up of both bed fund payments and casualty payments. The distribution of payments (which are superannuable) from this fund is agreed among the local participating doctors attached to the hospital. Only GPs on the Health Authority or Health Board list are appointed to the staff of a GP hospital under the bed fund arrangement, and they are free to organize for themselves how the work is undertaken. As independent clinicians they are accountable to their peers. The calculation of bed fund payments for inpatient GP beds is based on bed occupancy not time spent on the work.

Box 8.4: Key features of staff fund arrangements

- independent clinical responsibility – no consultant supervision
- doctor controls admission, management, administration and discharge
- no sick leave
- no study leave
- no annual leave
- no security of tenure
- no travel and other expenses
- very poorly paid

Casualty payments are paid into the bed fund and form part of it. The clinical assistant scale is used to calculate the size of these payments, but the payments as such are not connected to that grade. There are two kinds of payments: a retention fee and a fee which reflects the number of patient attendances. The fee based on attendance reflects the number of new patient attendances and the clinical assistant scale is normally used as an analogue for the rate of payments though this may vary locally.

Typically a given number of new attendances draws one clinical assistant session payment into the bed fund. Although the arrangements for casualty payments do not necessarily require GPs to see all patients when they first attend, each patient should be seen by a doctor at some stage. Nurses may treat minor problems, seeking advice and assistance from GPs as necessary. However, a GP must be available to attend immediately if required.

The content of a contract for hospital services

The contract should state to which consultant the GP is clinically responsible. If supervised by a consultant, the post should normally be graded as either clinical assistant or hospital practitioner; the latter may be preferred because it has greater security of tenure and is more highly paid. Contracts for both grades should specify hours of work; however, it should be noted that although it is comparatively easy to calculate sessional payments for routine work it is usually more difficult to do so for out-of-hours work.

The hours during which casualty work is to be covered must be clearly specified; some GPs with surgeries on the same site as a GP hospital have found that between 9 a.m. and 5 p.m. they receive no pay for casualty work because health authorities mistakenly consider it to be part of general medical services.

Box 8.5: Contract checklist

The contract should include:

- name of employing authority
- date employment commences and any previous employment which may count towards continuity
- place of work
- job description
- hours of work
- superannuation
- remuneration
- annual leave
- study leave
- maternity leave
- sick leave
- definition of clinical responsibility
- substitution and deputizing arrangements
- medical indemnity
- period of notice of termination
- disciplinary procedure
- grievance procedure
- reference to the terms and conditions of service for hospital medical and dental staff, as appropriate.

9 Flexible and Part-time Working in General Practice

> **Where to obtain advice and assistance**
>
> BMA members can obtain expert advice and assistance on all contractual problems from their local BMA office. Health Authorities are also an important source of advice. The BMA has published guidance on contracts for GP salaried assistants which includes a model contract of employment.
>
> Further reading includes Ellis N and Stanton T (eds) (1994) *Making Sense of Partnerships*. Radcliffe Medical Press, Oxford and Ellis N and Chisholm J (1997) *Making Sense of the Red Book*. Third edition, Radcliffe Medical Press, Oxford.

The main opportunities for flexible and part-time working in general practice are:

- as a principal, particularly part-time and job sharing GPs
- as a restricted services principal
- as a part-time salaried employee – often termed an assistant
- as a member of the doctors' retainer scheme
- as an associate
- as a locum.

Although there are important statutory regulations and employment law governing these flexible and part-time arrangements, the actual contractual terms are matters to be agreed between the practice and the doctor. This latter point is important and needs to be stressed; much of the advice provided below is drawn from the BMA's recommendations relating to fair and reasonable contractual terms, but cannot be regarded as mandatory.

Part-time working as a GP principal

Five options of availability

The GP's terms of service provide five options of availability to patients. These arrangements do not alter a GP's basic responsibility to ensure that, either personally or through a deputy, general medical services are provided for patients throughout each and every day that his or her name is included on a Health Authority or Health Board list.

Full-time over five days

This option requires a GP to be normally available for not less than 26 hours spread over five days each week, for 42 weeks in any 12-month period.

Full-time over four days

This second option allows a GP to be normally available for not less than 26 hours spread over four days each week for 42 weeks in any 12-month period. Doctors may apply for this option if they are involved in health-related activities, which are defined in the NHS regulations as those connected with:

- organization of the medical profession or training of its members
- providing medical care or treatment
- improving quality of care or treatment
- administering general medical services.

Health Authorities and Health Boards should be guided by the illustrative list of these activities shown in Box 9.1.

Three-quarter time

A three quarter time contract allows a GP to be normally available for not less than 19 hours each week on days to be agreed with the Health Authority or Health Board, for 42 weeks each year. This option is only available to GPs in a partnership with at least one full-time practitioner.

Half-time

A half time GP normally has to be available for not less than 13 hours each week on days to be agreed with the Health Authority or Health Board,

---

Box 9.1: Health related activities

- appointments concerned with medical education or training; for example, regional adviser, course organizer or an academic appointment

- medical appointments within the health service other than in relation to the provision of general medical services; for example, hospital appointments (such as hospital practitioner, clinical assistant and GP hospital posts) and also health service management and advisory posts, including Health Authority and Health Board duties

- medical appointments made under the Crown, with Government departments or agencies, or public or local authorities; for example, medical work for the police or prison service

- appointments concerning the regulation of the medical profession or the MPC; for example, General Medical Council (GMC) appointments, membership of the national GMSCs (including Welsh, Scottish and Northern Ireland GMSCs) or the Royal College of General Practitioners (RCGP) at national level, or service on an LMC

---

for 42 weeks each year. This option is only available to GPs in a partnership with at least one full-time practitioner.

Job sharing

This enables a joint application by doctors in a partnership which includes both of them. Together they must be normally available for not less than 26 hours over five days each week for 42 weeks each year. The two doctors should decide how the 26 hours are to be divided.

Non-availability

Each of the above options requires the GP to be normally available for 42 weeks in any 12-month period. Throughout the 42 weeks but outside approved hours and during the remaining 10 weeks, a GP is free to make reasonable arrangement with a partner or a deputy for the care of patients.

Box 9.2: Minimum profit shares of part-timers

Full-time principals	minimum share is one-third of that of partner with the greatest share
Three-quarter time principals	minimum share is one-quarter of that of partner with the greatest share
Half-time principals	minimum share is one-fifth of that of partner with the greatest share
Job sharers	minimum joint share is one-third of that of partner with greatest share

(These minimum profit shares apply only to the NHS component of the partnership profits. Income from work outside NHS general practice is excluded from the calculation.)

Profit share and part-time partners

Under NHS regulations, for the Health Authority or Health Board to recognize GPs as partners, it must be satisfied that they discharge the duties and exercise the powers of principals in the partnership and are entitled to a profit share based on one of the options in Box 9.2.

Each partnership must decide for itself how to run its business. But if any partner's share is grossly out of line with his or her contribution to the practice's workload, a concealed sale of goodwill may be deemed to have taken place.

Discrimination

It is unlawful for a partnership of two or more partners to discriminate on grounds of sex or marital status, and for a partnership of six or more partners to discriminate on grounds of colour, race, nationality (including citizenship) or ethnic or national origins:

- when appointing a new partner
- in the terms on which the new partner is offered a partnership
- by refusing, or deliberately neglecting to offer a partnership

and where someone is already a partner:

- in the way he or she is afforded access to any benefits, facilities or services
- by refusing, or deliberately neglecting, to afford access to those benefits, facilities and services
- by dismissing the partner, or treating him or her unfavourably in any other way.

Maternity leave

As self-employed independent contractors women GP principals do not enjoy the employment rights relating to pregnancy and childbirth that apply to women employees. Thus partnerships are free to make their own arrangements for an individual partner's maternity leave. (*See* Box 9.3 for an outline of some recommended maternity leave arrangements for partnerships.)

There are various arrangements for paying locums employed during prolonged absences such as those arising from sickness or maternity leave. A simple method is for the absent partner to pay all the locum expenses. However, it is increasingly common for the first few weeks of locum expenses to be paid by the whole partnership.

A partnership will be infringing the Sex Discrimination Act 1976 if a pregnant partner is treated less favourably than a male partner with a distinctly male incapacity. Therefore a partner on maternity leave should not have to meet the full cost of a locum unless this arrangement also applies to sick leave.

A woman GP who provides unrestricted general medical services and is paid a basic practice allowance can claim additional payments for a locum actually engaged during absences due to pregnancy and childbirth. These payments are similar to those paid during sickness, but for maternity there are no list size criteria. The payments are available for a maximum period of 14 weeks. These additional payments from the Health Authority or Health Board should be paid to the absent partner if she is responsible for locum expenses. (Eligibility for additional payments during sickness

---

Box 9.3: Recommended arrangements for maternity leave

- 14 weeks absence should be regarded as a minimum entitlement and the pregnant partner should have the right to determine for herself when the period of absence should start, in consultation with her own GP
- the practice should consider the question of funding the cost of a locum to cover the actual workload of the pregnant partner, not merely her hours of availability
- the partnership should agree on a maximum period of absence following which a partner's failure to return to work may justify compulsory expulsion
- the exercise of a partner's right to maternity leave should not abolish her entitlement to *pro rata* holiday and sickness leave
- where this seems appropriate the partnership agreement should specify leave arrangements for adoption

A partnership agreement which provides for maternity leave on terms which are less advantageous than sick leave could be construed as evidence of indirect sex discrimination.

---

depend on the average number of patients that the remaining GPs have to care for during the absence.)

The question of how long a partnership or individual partner pays locum expenses needs to be decided in relation to the arrangements for insurance cover for income protection and/or locum expenses.

Partnership agreements

As well as the minimum share of the profits referred to above, a doctor who is in partnership must discharge the duties and exercise the powers of a principal in the running of the partnership; irrespective of whether he or she is a part-time, job-sharing or full time principal.

Working as a restricted services principal

The 'restricted services principal' provides general medical services which are limited to:

- child health surveillance services

- contraceptive services
- maternity medical services
- minor surgery services
- or any combination of these.

This is quite distinct from the 'restricted list principal' who cares for a restricted category of patients connected with a particular establishment or organization.

In general, a restricted services principal is eligible to only receive:

- those fees related to the particular service being provided
- discretionary payments under the rent and rates scheme and practice staff scheme.

Restricted principals providing maternity, contraceptive or child health surveillance services are also eligible to receive modified payments under the sickness and confinement schemes; but those providing only minor surgery services are not.

Doctors applying to become restricted principals for the minor surgery and child health surveillance lists will be approved only if they work either in a group with one or more principals or as an assistant or deputy of a principal who is on the relevant list. A restricted services principal must satisfy the specific criteria for entry to the relevant special list.

Working as a salaried assistant

The GP's terms of service require the Health Authority or Health Board to be told when an assistant is being employed. The GP is not allowed to employ one or more assistants for more than three months in any 12-month period without Health Authority or Health Board consent, irrespective of whether the assistant's employment qualifies for the assistant's allowance.

GPs may employ assistants at their own expense; they are eligible for additional payments (the assistant's allowance) only if the criteria in Red Book paragraphs 18.1–18.6 are satisfied.

GPs are also eligible for additional payments for employing a locum to cover an assistant's absence because of sickness or maternity, if the assistant continues to be paid full salary during the period of absence.

Assistants should agree with their employing practices written contracts and job descriptions. Every employer is required to issue a written statement of the main terms of employment to any employee working at least eight hours per week within two months of starting work.

Anyone considering working as an assistant may find the following checklist a helpful guide to those subjects which should be covered by an employment contract:

• pay including provision for annual review
• hours of work including any flexibility requirement
• holiday leave and pay entitlement
• sick leave and pay entitlement
• maternity leave and pay entitlement
• pensions arrangements
• notice of termination of contract
• grievance procedures
• arrangements for motoring expenses, medical defence organization and other professional subscriptions.

In addition, there should be an agreed job description which describes the post's responsibilities and duties. Box 9.4 summarizes the employment rights of part-timers and whole-timers.

GP assistant's pay

It is not possible to specify a particular rate of pay or formula for determining pay which can suit all circumstances; ultimately a GP assistant's salary has to reflect the circumstances of the appointment: relevant factors include previous experience, hours of work, job content and the income of the practice. The GMSC has suggested two possible ways of determining a GP assistant's salary:

• a specific rate of pay such as a salary which may be linked to some external comparator
• a formula which relates pay to the income of the practice.

Whichever is used, the actual salary must take account of both the practice's financial circumstances and the nature of the post itself.

The option of basing an assistant's salary on a specific rate of pay has the advantage of simplicity (possible analogues include the NHS clinical assistant and hospital practitioner grades). The actual pay rate could take account of various factors including:

• previous experience
• hours of work

Box 9.4: Part-timers' employment rights

Minimum weekly hours and length of service required to qualify for statutory employment rights are set out below. These employment rights were introduced under the Employment Protection (part-time employees) Regulations 1995 (SI 1995/31).

Employment right	under eight hours	eight hours or more
Unfair dismissal (general)	no right	two years' service
Unfair dismissal (inadmissible reasons)	unrestricted	unrestricted
Notice of dismissal	no right	one month's service
Written reason for dismissal[a]	no right	two years' service
Redundancy pay	no right	two years' service
Right to return after maternity absence (up to 29 weeks after childbirth)	no right	two years' service
Maternity leave (14 weeks)[b]	unrestricted	unrestricted
Statutory maternity pay[c]	no right	six months' service (see footnote)
Written particulars	no right	two months' service
Guaranteed pay	no right	two years' service
Time off for union duties	no right	unrestricted
Equal pay	unrestricted	unrestricted
Sex discrimination	unrestricted	unrestricted
Race discrimination	unrestricted	unrestricted
Ante-natal leave	unrestricted	unrestricted

[a] If a woman is pregnant or taking maternity leave when dismissed, the right to written reasons is unrestricted by service requirements.

[b] Various new maternity rights introduced by the Trade Union Reform and Employment Rights Act 1993 come into force in October 1994. A woman is eligible to take 40 weeks' maternity leave if she works at least 16 hours a week and has at least 2 years' service (or between eight and 16 hours and five years' service).

[c] SMP is paid after six months; entitlement to higher rate SMP (90 percent of earnings) depends on length of service and hours worked per week.

- out-of-hours commitment
- duties performed.

Some practices may wish to use a fairly complex formula to calculate relative workloads of both partners and salaried assistants.

The other option, where an assistant's salary is based on a percentage of practice profits, also needs to take account of the factors listed above. It is hard to specify a percentage of parity to suit all circumstances; the GMSC has suggested that a minimum 70–75% of parity should be a fair basis for calculating the salary for a full time GP assistant who does the whole range of general medical service duties (including the practice's out-of-hours commitment) but does not share the managerial responsibilities of the employing partners.

The doctors' retainer scheme

The scheme helps doctors under the age of 55 years who work not more than one day a week to keep in touch with medicine so that they can return to the NHS when circumstances permit. They are offered the opportunity of doing a small amount of paid professional work and to attend postgraduate medical education sessions; in return, scheme members are paid a retainer to help meet expenses. Some 600 GPs are currently in the scheme.

A doctor joining the scheme agrees to:

- maintain GMC registration and membership of a medical defence organization
- attend at least seven educational sessions a year, which may be arranged to fit in with family responsibilities
- take a professional journal such as the *British Medical Journal*
- work at least one half-day a month and be prepared to take on more work, up to maximum of one day a week (if asked to do so) if this does not interfere with family commitments.

How the scheme is organized

Health Authorities have been responsible for the general administration of the scheme; they accept new members and pay the annual retainer fee. Professional advice and guidance about educational facilities are provided by clinical tutors who should discuss career prospects with scheme members and advise them on local postgraduate activities. Clinical tutors review progress with scheme members at least annually. Educational sessions attended by members should be relevant to their current work and their eventual return to regular practice.

Scheme members may work in various fields; including hospitals, general practice, public health medicine and community health services. The employer is responsible for arranging and paying for work done. Membership is on a year by year basis and continues automatically for a whole year even if a member's professional commitments increase to more than one day a week.

The retainer fee and income tax

The retainer fee should be treated as earned income and taxed under Schedule E; but it is not liable for superannuation or NI contributions. After deducting allowable expenses, the remaining balance will attract any personal income tax relief to which the doctor is entitled; these expenses are those incurred wholly exclusively, and necessarily, in the performance of professional duties; for example, the annual GMC retention fee and subscriptions to professional bodies, such as a medical defence organization and the BMA. (Subscription rates to medical defence organizations and the BMA are reduced for doctors with this level of income.)

Other fees: superannuation and income tax

Although fees paid by the practice for work done under the scheme are liable to income tax and class 1 NI contributions, they are not superannuable even if the retainee is described as an assistant. However, if a doctor already has two or more years service with the NHS Pension Scheme his or her accrued benefits can be preserved. If total service is less than this, these benefits may be lost after a 12-month break in service; the doctor can prevent this by working at least one day in each 12-month period in superannuable employment. Alternatively if none of the work undertaken in connection with the scheme is superannuable (e.g. working as a GP assistant) a doctor may apply to the NHS Pensions Agency at the Department of Health, 200–220 Broadway, Fleetwood, Lancs FY7 8LG, for employment under the scheme to be 'approved' for superannuation purposes, in order to avoid incurring a disqualifying break in service of 12 months or more.

At the time of writing the Department of Health has agreed to a revision of the Scheme. The GMSC is currently formulating a new package.

Working as an associate

The Associate scheme enables single-handed isolated GPs to employ an associate. This allows them regular time off and training, in circumstances where continuous duty is an otherwise inescapable feature of their practice. Normally an associate is employed by two practices; although three may sometimes be appropriate. (GPs with assistants are ineligible for the scheme.)

Those GPs who participate in this scheme, and are also paid inducement payments, are no longer entitled to claim locum expenses, other than in the most exceptional circumstances.

Box 9.5 explains how the scheme has been modified to take account of the special geographical circumstances of remote areas of Scotland.

Box 9.5: Special Scottish circumstances

Particular geographical difficulties, especially in the highlands and islands, may mean that it is impractical for two or three neighbouring principals to employ an associate. In these circumstances, Health Boards can organize a scheme if asked to do so by GPs.

GPs in very isolated areas, where groupings of two or three eligible principals are difficult if not impossible to arrange, can ask their Health Board to act as the paying agent on their behalf and to employ a suitably qualified associate. Though the Board appoints, pays and deploys these associates, responsibility for them under the terms of service remains with the principal. In these circumstances, where the Board only acts solely as the agent, GPs should ensure that they are adequately represented on the selection panel appointed by the Board to recruit associates.

To qualify for this allowance a GP must be single-handed (including job sharers) and:

• in receipt of rural practice payments

OR

- the sole practitioner on an island

AND ALSO

- in receipt of an inducement payment

OR

- practising more than 10 miles (measured along the most practicable route) from the nearest GP's main surgery or nearest district general hospital.

Doctors employed as associates must satisfy vocational training regulations and be eligible to apply to join an Health Authority or Health Board list, but whilst holding this appointment must not be included on such a list.

Associates undertake all GP work and their employing GPs are responsible for their actions including any breach of the terms of service. The associate scheme is broadly similar to the GP trainee scheme; the associate doctor has the same contractual relationship with the GP employer, the same accountability arrangements and the same tax status as a trainee does.

Because a GP principal is accountable for the activities of an associate, he or she should employ someone with the necessary skills and aptitude to be able to practise in social and professional isolation. This scheme may become a step in the career structure, offering a route to obtaining an isolated or inducement practice. A short-term 'apprenticeship' as an associate can enable a younger doctor to assess his or her own suitability for this type of practice.

The employing practice decides the associate's salary, but the amount reimbursed directly by the Health Authority or Health Board will be on the associate scale of payments as set annually by the Review Body. Other reimbursements include a car allowance, telephone expenses, removal expenses, the cost of medical defence organization subscriptions, the employer's NI contributions and other expenses similar to those covered by the GP trainee practitioner scheme. An associate may receive the postgraduate education allowance and time spent as an associate will count towards seniority payments in the same way as for GP assistants. Where two or three GPs jointly employ an associate, one of them has to be responsible to the Health Authority or Health Board for administering salary, allowances and tax deductions.

The Health Authority or Health Board has to be satisfied that the arrangements ensure continuity of care for patients, equitable and regular time off for both the GPs and the associate, that they cover the annual and postgraduate study leave, and that the associate is employed on a full time basis. (In England and Wales the Health Authority can ask to see the associate's contract of employment.)

What an associate does

It is for the employing doctors to determine how an associate is deployed between the participating practices. However, doctors in isolated areas often have small lists of a few hundred patients so it is inappropriate for a principal to use the associate as simply an extra pair of hands; it is not the practice's workload that should need relieving but the unremitting on-call commitment. Most participating GPs will wish to be relieved of their practice responsibilities on a regular basis (probably for at least a week at a time) to compensate for the difficulties of ferry travel or long road journeys when leaving the practice area for a worthwhile break. At other times (e.g. school holidays) it should be possible to arrange a sustained break whilst staying in their own area knowing that time with their families will not be disrupted by practice commitments. It should be remembered that any practice arrangements will be subject to disruption in the event of sickness or maternity leave involving either practitioner or associate. When this occurs, balancing periods of leave or extra duty may be required to ensure equity.

Working as a locum

Locums in general practice can work long term or short term, part-time or full-time to cover, for example, a principal's absence on maternity or study leave, extended leave of absence or illness, or to cover a period before a new partner is appointed. Terms of employment vary, as does the existence of a contract of employment. Some locums also work for deputizing services on a sessional basis.

Doctors may find locum employment advantageous, say, following vocational training when they may want experience in various practices before becoming a principal. Disadvantages may include poor job satisfaction, especially when there is no opportunity for continuity of patient care, lack of a proper contract of employment, poor pay and inadequate continuing medical education. Only long-term locums are eligible to claim Section 63 expenses for travel and subsistence to attend educational courses. Expenses are not normally reimbursed for locums on short-term contracts. The BMA can advise members on appropriate fees for locum work.

10 Part-time Medical Work Outside the NHS

Where to obtain advice and assistance

BMA members can obtain expert advice and assistance from their local BMA office. The BMA's Private Practice and Professional Fees Committee negotiates or suggests fees for almost all part-time services GPs undertake outside their main NHS contract. GP members are sent annually a pocket size BMA fees guide which gives information on the most frequently claimed fees. The BMA also provides free to members a general guidance note on *Fees for part-time medical services* and its various supplements give up-to-date information on the suggested negotiated and statutory fees. All matters concerning occupational health are looked after by the BMA's Occupational Health Committee. It publishes a comprehensive booklet *The Occupational Physician* which is available to BMA members free of charge.

Further reading includes Locke C (1994) *Private Medical Practice*. Radcliffe Medical Press, Oxford.

Although there are no official data on the amount of non-NHS work GPs undertake, unpublished data and anecdotal evidence suggest that the totality of GPs' earnings from this source amounts on average to barely one or two per cent of their gross NHS income. Thus the total amount of these earnings is probably much smaller than is generally assumed. The extent of this work within general practice is often overestimated, because a small minority of practices who are heavily and enthusiastically involved in it have given wide publicity to its considerable potential income.

The main sources of GP earnings outside the NHS are:

- a wide range of miscellaneous fees paid for various part-time medical services
- private general practice
- work in occupational health.

Non-NHS medical work

GPs may charge fees for a range of non-NHS work, including fees for local or central government work, reports or certificates for their patients or third parties and private treatment. Nevertheless, it needs to be remembered that GPs are prohibited by their NHS contracts from charging fees in certain specific circumstances (*see* Box 3.9, Chapter 3).

The level of fees that may be charged depends on whom the work is being carried out for and how the level is determined. The BMA divides these fees into four main categories (designated A, B, C and D) according to how they are determined (*see* Box 10.1).

Box 10.1: BMA categories of fees

Category A	fees prescribed by statute
Category B	fee negotiated nationally by the BMA with Government departments, local authorities and other employers
Category C	fees negotiated nationally with representative bodies
Category D	fee suggested by the BMA

The BMA publishes 12 fees guidance schedules (*see* Box 10.2) which describe the level of fees applying to a particular area of work and the circumstances in which they may be paid; these cover several hundred individual fees and help to ensure GPs are paid correctly for their non-NHS services. The fees guidance supplements are only available to BMA members, free of charge, from their local BMA office.

The BMA considers that if an official body commissions a medical examination, report or certificate for which a GP may charge a fee, it should be liable for meeting the costs.

Box 10.2: Fees guidance schedules

The following fees guidance schedules are available separately from local BMA offices:

FGS1   Central government departments and agencies
FGS2   Work for local health authorities
FGS3   Sessional and miscellaneous work in the NHS
FGS4   Family planning
FGS5   Life assurance work
FGS6   Charitable societies
FGS7   Road accidents: emergency treatment
FGS8   Police work
FGS9   Work for coroners and crematoria
FGS10   Medico-legal fees
FGS11   Where no agreement applies
FGS12   Medical cover in general practice

Category A: statutory fees

A typical example is the fee for providing emergency treatment at road traffic accidents. These fees are always paid strictly according to the conditions stipulated in the relevant legislation. Box 10.3 lists the main types of fees in this category.

Category B: fees negotiated with central government departments and public sector employers

These are traditionally linked to Review Body recommendations; typical examples include fees for part-time services to certain government departments, local authorities and police authorities. They are paid by the government department or employer which negotiated the fee. Box 10.4 summarizes the main fees in this category. At the time of writing the profession is in dispute with various government departments because they have deliberately breached an agreement to increase these fees.

Box 10.3: Category A: statutory fees and fees determined by government departments

- fees for blood tests and reports relating to evidence of paternity
- allowances to witnesses to fact in criminal cases for both written medical reports and attendance at court (FGS10)
- emergency treatment at road traffic accidents (FGS7)
- examinations under the Factories Acts and health and safety at work legislation
- medical examinations required under the diving regulations
- aviation medical fees
- dental anaesthetic fees
- seafarers' statutory medical examinations

Category C: fees negotiated with representative organizations

Typical examples are fees for life assurance reports, and work for voluntary and charitable societies. The BMA's negotiated fees apply to only those organizations which are members of the national representative body; for example, life assurance report fees are only binding on member companies of the British Association of Life Insurers. Box 10.5 lists the main fees in this category.

Category D: suggested fees

This category includes all those fees not determined by negotiation or statute; they are left to be agreed between the GP and the party concerned. The extensive list of the many and varied types in Box 10.6 is provided as a reminder of private service for which GPs may charge patients. GPs are often reticent about charging NHS patients for non-NHS services and patients are correspondingly reluctant to pay for them. In a publicly funded service which is still permeated by the non-pecuniary ethos, GPs and patients are unaccustomed to monetary transactions. Each practice will obviously determine its own policy on charging patients for this work; a determined effort may have to be made to overcome any inhibitions about introducing the cash nexus into patient-doctor relations, and to inform patients of which NHS service they can legitimately expect to receive free of charge, and for which non-NHS services they can properly be charged.

Box 10.4: Category B: work for central government departments

Range of fees for various procedures including:

- medical examinations and reports
- medical attendance on non-NHS patients
- regular attendance at government establishments

Employment Service Division

- disablement advisory committees panels

Department of Transport

- extract from medical records or completing DVLA question-naires
- DVLA diagnostic tests

DSS

- fees for various reports required for pension and other purposes
- part-time referee for the Benefits Agency medical service
- membership of various tribunals

HSE

- extracts from records plus opinion

Home Office (Prison Service)

- part-time prison medical officers (agreed directly with the Home Office (Prison Service)

Box 10.5: Category C: fees for private sector work

- fees for life assurance reports (FGS5)
- voluntary aid societies (e.g. British Red Cross Society, St John Ambulance Association) (FGS6)

Box 10.6: Category D: fees suggested by the BMA for various types of private work

(Most of these fees are covered by FGS11)

- holiday insurance certificate
- blood test (not involving disputed paternity)
- court of protection medical certificates
- cervical cytology (non-NHS)
- private medical consultations
- copying medical notes
- comprehensive medical examinations and reports
- fitness to attend court as a witness
- cremation forms B and C
- removal of a pacemaker following death
- pre-employment examinations
- reports requested by employers
- private sickness absence certificates for school or work
- motor insurance certificates of fitness
- accident and sickness insurance certificates
- validation of provident association claim form
- school fees insurance
- fitness for higher education
- fitness to participate in a sport
- freedom from infection certificate
- vaccination and immunization
- attendances at police stations not covered by NHS fee at patient's request
- family planning
- lecture fees
- non-NHS minor surgery
- seatbelt exemption certificates
- prescriptions for drugs required in overseas travel
- reports for drug companies

continued opposite

Box 10.6: *continued*

- race meetings and sporting activities
- private nursing homes
- data protection legislation: search of records
- access to medical records: copying fee
- reports on prospective subscribers to health insurance
- non-medical services (e.g. passport signing)
- payments to deputizing doctors
- fees for involvement in legal work (i.e. professional witnesses and expert witnesses where legal aid does not apply)

Deciding what to charge

GPs should clarify whether they are entitled to charge a fee before agreeing to provide a service. If it is clear that a fee may be charged, the next question that has to be answered is for whom is the medical service being provided. This is crucial because its answer determines both the level of fee and who should pay it. Whether or not a fee may be charged is determined by either statute or the GP's terms of service. It is advisable to forewarn patients of any charge before undertaking the work. Hopefully this should avoid some of the embarrassment that can arise in NHS general practice when charges are being made for non-NHS services. Some practices find it helpful to have a notice about this in the waiting room.

GPs are obliged under paragraph 13 of their terms of service to provide patients with 'all necessary and appropriate personal medical services of the type usually provided by general practitioners' for which they are not permitted to ask or accept, any payment (*see* paragraph 37) except if this is specifically allowed in the terms of service (*see* paragraph 38). A full list of services for which an NHS patient may be charged is in Box 3.9 (Chapter 3). Although some certificates may be charged for, NHS GPs are obliged under the terms of service to provide the certificates specified in Box 3.9 (Chapter 3) free of charge, including those supporting social security benefit claims.

Private general practice

There is no limit on the amount of private practice NHS GPs may undertake provided they fulfil their NHS commitment. If staff or premises, which are directly reimbursed for NHS purposes, are used and a practice's private practice income is more than 10 per cent of total practice receipts, these NHS reimbursements will be proportionally abated. Under no circumstances, except those referred to above which are permitted under their terms of service, can GPs charge a fee to their own NHS patients.

The actual amount of private practice undertaken by NHS GPs as a whole is very small; only a small minority of practices are likely to have a significant number of private patients. Typically NHS GPs accept private patients only on request; they do not advertise for patients, though they are now free to do so subject to the guidance laid down by the General Medical Council.

An NHS GP cannot treat a patient both privately and on the NHS concurrently. This is because GPs' terms of service prohibit them from accepting any payment from patients for whose treatment they are responsible under their NHS contract, unless such payments are specifically authorized. This restriction on receiving payments extends to patients registered with the GP's partners. Some patients have both an NHS GP and a private GP from a different practice.

A private GP may agree to be 'on call' for private patients but is not obliged to do so unless the contract with the patient specifically includes an out-of-hours service. The NHS out-of-hours contractual obligation does not apply to the private sector.

NHS GPs must only provide an NHS prescription (FP10) to their NHS patients; they cannot prescribe an NHS prescription for private patients.

Many NHS GPs treat their private patients on the same or a similar basis to their NHS patients; both surgery and domiciliary consultations are arranged to fit in with their NHS commitments.

Private general practice is based on a personal contract between the doctor and patient. For some years the provident associations have not shown any interest in offering insurance schemes to cover the costs of private general practice, although some insurance companies have recently expressed an interest in such policies.

There is one aspect of general practice which merits further clarification, namely the treatment of overseas visitors. The Health Department circular which governs these matters (HN(FP)(84)7) states that, apart from immediately necessary (i.e. emergency) treatment, the NHS GP has unrestricted discretion as to whether to treat a non-EU visitor as a temporary resident and NHS patient, or as a wholly private patient. The health circular makes it clear that many non-EU visitors expect to pay for medical treatment and GPs will not be committing any offence or breach of their terms of service if they offer to treat overseas visitors privately on whatever terms are mutually agreed. However, most visitors from other EU countries have some

Box 10.7: Services for which fees may not be charged

Death certificates

In England and Wales, the registered medical practitioner who was in attendance upon the deceased during his or her last illness must deliver a death certificate, stating to the best of his or her knowledge and belief, the cause of death to the local registrar forthwith, and he or she may not charge a fee for this service. Failure to deliver the certificate 'without reasonable excuse' is punishable on summary conviction with a fine. He or she must also hand the person designated as 'qualified informant' the outer detachable part of the certificate form entitled 'Notice to Informant', duly completed.

Stillbirth certificates

Any registered medical practitioner who was present at the birth or examined the body of a stillborn child must, upon a request from the 'qualified informant', give a certificate stating that the child was not born alive, and, where possible, stating to the best of his or her knowledge and belief the cause of death and estimated duration of the pregnancy.

GPs under contract to Health Authorities (Health Board in Scotland)

The items for which doctors may not make charges are listed in Schedule 2 (term of service for doctors) of the NHS (General Medical Services) Regulations 1992 (Statutory Instrument No 635) as amended. In Scotland they are listed in Schedule 1 of The NHS (General Medical and Pharmaceutical Services) (Scotland) Regulations 1974 (Statutory Instrument No 506) as amended. Subsequent amendments are incorporated into the following:

(i)   England and Wales   Paragraphs 38–42 of the England and Wales Schedule

(ii) Scotland   Paragraph 20 of the Scottish Schedule.

entitlement under EU regulations to use the NHS, including GP services. Their entitlement varies according to their employment and/or visitor status. For most purposes it is best to assume they (together with nationals from non-EU or European Economic Area states who have signed the European Social Charter) are entitled to free NHS treatment, except in the case of treatment which they have specifically come to the UK to obtain.

The circular also states that if no local NHS GP is willing to treat the non-EU visitor on an NHS basis, he or she can apply to the Health Authority to be assigned to the list of a local GP. The GP to whom the patient is assigned is obliged to provide NHS general medical services free of charge for the minimum number of days as specified in the NHS terms of service. There is, however, a major difference between primary and secondary care. Even if an overseas visitor receives NHS general medical services, access to NHS secondary care entirely depends upon residency status and country of origin.

Occupational health

Although many doctors working in this specialty hold full-time salaried posts in large commercial and industrial organizations, there are also many part-time occupational physicians, most of whom are GPs. Some small firms prefer to employ a local doctor on a part-time sessional basis and GPs are ideally suited to fill these posts, although many firms have no occupational health service at all.

The BMA's Occupational Health Committee publishes suggested salary ranges for full and part-time occupational physician posts and annualized salaries based on one hour, two hours or one session (three and a half hours) per week. These scales are included in a BMA booklet *The Occupational Physician* which also provides guidance on managing occupational health departments, and notes on health and safety in the workplace. These scales take account of the doctor's qualifications in occupational medicine (e.g. AFOM or DIH), previous relevant experience and level of responsibility. Thus GPs who are members or fellows of the Faculty of Occupational Medicine and are accredited specialists and/or have considerable experience should start at relatively higher salaries. The scales are based on the assumption that the GP does not benefit from paid annual leave or membership of the firm's superannuation scheme.

An occupational physician is in a somewhat unusual position in relation to the organization's workforce in that there may be a danger that the normal rules governing medical ethics and confidentiality conflict with his or her responsibility to the organization's management. Guidance on how

---

Box 10.8: The duties of an occupational physician are of two main kinds:

- assessing and moderating the effects of health on an individual's capacity to work, including:
  - advising employers on such matters as pre-employment and annual medical examinations
  - immediately treating clinical emergencies at the place of work
  - examining and monitoring employees returning to work after prolonged sickness absence
  - advising management on health surveillance and screening
- assessing and moderating the effects of work on an individual's health which includes:
  - providing first aid services
  - examining and supervising medically those employees exposed to special hazards
  - advising management on the working environment, health risks, safety hazards and statutory requirements relating to health and safety at the workplace
  - supervising the hygiene of staff facilities, especially kitchens, canteens etc
  - educating the staff on matters pertaining to health, fitness and hygiene.

---

to handle these potentially conflicting responsibilities is provided in two BMA publications *The Occupational Physician* and *Medical Ethics Today: its philosophy and practice.*

Police surgeon work

The remuneration of police surgeons (which is classified as category B work) consists of a flat rate 'availability fee' plus a two-tier item of service fee; the fee for the first case being higher than for subsequent cases on the same call-out. These item of service fees are also payable if a doctor who is not a contracted police surgeon agrees to undertake the police visit. The fees are jointly negotiated by the BMA and the local government employers' organization and apply throughout Great Britain.

The 'availability fee' is a standard flat rate payment and not dependent on fee income. It may be supplemented by a further payment if the doctor has a relevant qualification (e.g. the diploma of medical jurisprudence or some other recognized qualification in forensic medicine) or has had 15 years' continuous service as a police surgeon (or deputy), normally with the same police force.

The item of service fees are paid when a doctor attends in response to a call from the police; they vary according to:

- when the call-out occurred
- length of time involved
- type of work undertaken
- whether a full written report or statement is required.

The work itself involves a varied range of duties, including:

- attending a police station to examine a prisoner, victim or police officer in relation to a wide variety of criminal offences
- occasional occupational health duties for the police force itself
- attending a scene of unexpected death to advise the police
- attending a court as a witness.

Future prospects

Radical changes in the way in which government departments contract for part-time medical services are in the offing, and these are creating a climate of uncertainty among GPs (and other doctors) who have traditionally undertaken this work. The life assurance industry is also reviewing its methods of assessing risks and questioning the value of the medical examination and report.

There are no signs of any general expansion in the demand for private general practice. Like other activities, this is affected by the economic climate and its prevalence is strongly influenced by specific local socioeconomic and cultural factors. It is heavily concentrated in particular localities where there is a predominance of foreign residents and patients with high disposable incomes.

The prospects for non-NHS part-time work for GPs are not favourable. The current economic climate has taken its toll on the opportunities for work in occupational medicine by bringing in its wake contractions and closures among many small businesses. Other firms have merged and rationalized their arrangements for occupational health medicine. However, more extensive and stringent health and safety laws may generate some expansion in this work.

11 Practice Accounts

The majority of GPs work in partnerships and almost all new GP principals enter general practice by joining an existing partnership. This chapter concentrates on the basic principles of accounting as they apply to partnerships. However, the basic accounting principles and methodology described below obviously apply equally to single-handed practitioners.

Partnership accounts provide a crucial record of a practice's profit for the accounting year and also show its financial worth at the balance sheet date. They also provide the Inland Revenue with information on which to assess the tax due from the partnership. Most importantly, the accounts should enable partners to review their practice's performance and plan its future development. They must, therefore, summarize clearly and concisely the practice's income and expenses and its net worth, and provide enough information to analyse its performance, including making comparisons with GPs' intended average gross and average net remuneration.

The income and expenditure account

This summarizes income – including investment income – and expenditure for the year. It is helpful to include the previous year's figures as comparatives so that partners can readily compare these with this year's performance. The following principles should be followed when preparing partnership accounts.

The grossing-up principle

As the Review Body pay award takes account of the level of expenses shown in GPs' accounts, together with personal claims for expenses and business interest relief included in their tax returns, it is important that all expenses are shown gross in the accounts. The NHS General Medical Services Statement of Fees and Allowances (the Red Book) advises that all income and expenses should be shown gross in the accounts, and that, for example, staff costs should not be netted off against staff reimbursements, or premises costs against rent and rates reimbursements.

The accruals basis

The income and expenditure account should be prepared on an accruals basis, i.e. in a way which reflects actual income earned and expenditure incurred during the accounting period, rather than simply cash paid and received. This is particularly relevant to any partnership where there has been a change of partners or profit shares; in these circumstances it is essential that all income earned and expenditure incurred by the partners in the year is allocated between them in that year's accounts. The term 'debtors' refers to the amount of money due to the practice at the balance sheet date; this consists mainly of Health Authority payments due to the practice at the end of the accounting year. For example, if the accounting year ends on 30th June, any fees and allowances received in the September quarter payment, which nevertheless relate to money earned during the June quarter, should be included as debtors.

DRS SMITH & PARTNERS
INCOME AND EXPENDITURE ACCOUNT
YEAR ENDED 30 JUNE 1996

	1996		1995	
	£	£	£	£
Income				
National Health Service fees	211 961		176 925	
Reimbursements	148 511		108 985	
Appointments	10 151		12 866	
Other income	10 113		7471	
Fundholding management allowance	24 916		12 646	
Total income		405 652		318 893
Expenditure				
Practice expenses	21 269		17 760	
Premises expenses	8359		6857	
Staff expenses	132 956		102 977	
Administration expenses	14 622		11 206	
Finance expenses	17 519		20 355	
Depreciation	2311		1178	
Fundholding expenses	24 916		11 168	
Total expenditure		221 952		171 501
		183 700		147 392
Investment income				
Bank interest receivable	766		211	
Building society interest receivable	1722		2101	
		2488		2312
Net profit for the year		186 188		149 704

Allocation of profits

	Prior shares £	Share of balance £	1996 Total £	1995 Total £
Dr Smith	11 063	38 241	49 304	41 603
Dr Patel	10 814	38 240	49 054	41 056
Dr Green	6523	38 240	44 763	35 428
Dr Jones	6791	36 276	43 067	31 617
	35 191	150 997	186 188	149 704

Figure 11.1 A sample income and expenditure account, showing allocation of profits

Valuing drugs

A stock-take needs to be made at the end of the accounting year of all drugs held by the practice. These should be valued at either cost or net realizable value, whichever is lower. Their value should be included on the balance sheet as an asset, being a part of the practice's net worth. Thus, if a partner retires from the practice, he or she has a share in the practice's stock of drugs, as valued at the end of the accounting year.

Depreciation

This charge is included in the income and expenditure account to enable the original cost of an asset to be spread over its useful life. The appropriate proportion of the original cost of an asset should be included in the expenses for each year, rather than reducing the profit of the year by the whole amount of its original cost. The partners (on the advice of their accountants) should decide which depreciation rates to apply to their assets. Once these have been decided they should be applied consistently. The following depreciation rates are commonly used:

- computer equipment $33\frac{1}{3}\%$ per annum
- medical equipment   20% per annum
- furniture and fittings   10% per annum
- office equipment   20% per annum
- motor cars   25% per annum
- surgery premises   not normally depreciated.

Since practices, or their accountants, can choose their own depreciation rates, the Inland Revenue does not give tax relief on the amount of depreciation included in the accounts. Instead, it allows tax relief on the purchase of fixed assets by means of standardized capital allowances.

Allocating profits to partners

When the profit for the accounting period has been calculated, it is then distributed among the partners according to the practice's profit sharing arrangements. If there are no changes in either the partnership or its profit sharing ratios during the year, this should be a comparatively straight-forward exercise. However, if such changes have occurred, it is necessary to allocate the profit by reference to the various profit sharing periods. This may be done by attempting to allocate it accurately between different profit sharing periods, such that income earned and expenditure incurred in these periods is identified and attributed to the relevant periods. This is, however, very time consuming and consequently, expensive to do. Alternatively, profits may be apportioned on a time basis, which means that if a new partner is admitted half-way through a year, half of the profits would be allocated to the first period and half to the second. This is the most popular method of distributing profits.

Obviously if the appointment or retirement of a partner is likely to affect significantly the practice's profitability, it may be advisable to apportion the income on a best estimate of the actual basis. However, because it is often extremely difficult to allocate expenses on a strictly actual basis, it may be fairer (and certainly much simpler) to apportion expenses on a time basis.

In principle, all items of practice income and expenditure must be included in the accounts so that the profit accurately reflects what is actually being generated by the practice. However, some practices have agreed that not all income should be shared among the partners according to their profit sharing ratios. Instead, income from sources such as seniority awards, night visit fees and postgraduate education allowance may be retained on a personal basis by individual partners. According to this arrangement, such income should be regarded as prior shares of profit and, therefore, allocated to partners before the resulting balance is divided between them according to the agreed profit sharing ratios. Similarly, if not all partners own the premises, or partners own the premises in different ratios to those applying to profit shares, income and expenditure relating to ownership of the surgery should be allocated as a prior share among property owning partners according to the ratios in which they own the premises. The net surgery income comprises Health Authority rent allowances less interest on partnership loans relating to the premises, and any other expenditure which it is agreed should be borne by the property owning partners.

Capital grants

If Health Authority improvement grants and fundholding management allowances are paid to a practice as a contribution towards its capital expenditure, these should be offset in the accounts against the cost of relevant assets so that only the net cost is depreciated and included in the balance sheet.

Health Authority improvement grant payments and fundholding management allowances need to be shown separately; although capital allowances may be claimed if a management allowance is paid, these cannot be claimed if an improvement grant is paid towards the cost of an asset. Any claim is additionally restricted to the net cost after reimbursement of the asset.

Presenting the accounts

Figure 11.1 shows an example of how to lay out income and expenditure accounts for a GP practice and how to allocate profits among partners. The accounts refer partners to more detailed information so that they can analyse the practice's performance. The various NHS fees and allowances received by the practice are shown in Figure 11.2.

The practice's income consists of four main elements: allowances, capitation payments, sessional payments and item of service fees. On average, a GP's income is distributed among these as follows:

- allowances   17%
- capitation payments   63%
- sessional payments   4%
- item of service payments   16%
  Total   100%

Practices should review how their income is distributed. A significant variation from the above pattern may point to areas where a practice can increase activity and income.

GPs are self-employed individuals for tax purposes and enter into a contract for services with their Health Authorities. The Review Body's pay award sets the levels of various NHS fees and allowances for the year. It also determines the intended average gross remuneration and the element of that gross income which is deemed to cover indirect expenses, thereby arriving at a figure for intended average net remuneration. The intended gross and net income per principal as set by the Review Body are published in the medical press, and practices should compare their accounts with these intended average levels.

Direct reimbursement

In addition to receiving indirect reimbursements for general expenses through the generality of fees and allowances, GPs are also directly reimbursed for practice staff, surgery premises, computers, drugs, trainee salaries, staff training and certain locum fees. It is also possible in certain cases to claim an allowance for the employment of an assistant or retained doctor. It is important that these direct reimbursements are shown clearly in the accounts so that a practice can identify easily the real cost of various activities; for example, the real cost of taking on an additional member of staff is the total cost less any direct reimbursement. In general, it is essential that direct reimbursements are not netted out against expenditure, because this reduces the total amount of expenses reported to the Review Body to enable it to determine GPs' pay.

Accounting records

The information in the income and expenditure account is obtained by the practice's accountants from the practice's own accounting records. These should comprise a cash book, a petty cash book, and an analysis of Health Authority income. The latter should show all fees and allowances received from the Health Authority during the year, dividing them into the elements shown in Figure 11.2. This provides a vital record for the practice to monitor NHS income and quickly identify any fall below the expected level.

The balance sheet

This is a statement of the practice's financial position at the end of the accounting year. It is important to note that it is merely a snap-shot of the amounts owed to and by the practice at a particular point in time. On the very next day cash may be received from a debtor, thereby increasing the amount shown as cash and reducing that shown as debtors, and in turn this cash may be used to pay a creditor. Such cash movements would not affect the practice's overall total net assets although these will change during the following year as profit is earned and drawn by partners.

The balance sheet has two distinct purposes: firstly, to ascertain whether the assets of the practice are sufficient to cover its liabilities and secondly to calculate the value of the partners' investment in the practice.

It is important to recognize that the accounts being prepared are those of the business in its own right and not those of its owners, who are the partners. This is an important distinction; these have to be seen as separate entities if their relationship (which is clearly shown in the balance sheet) is to be properly understood. Partners invest their funds in the practice as a business and therefore the balance sheet shows in the capital and current

National health service fees	1996 £	1995 £
Allowances		
Practice allowances	22 835	21 732
Seniority awards	4900	3523
Postgraduate education allowances	8100	7727
Rural practice payments	428	308
Trainee supervision grant	4237	4021
Out-of-hours allowances	4000	–
	44 500	37 311
Capitation payments		
Capitation fees	94 237	83 673
Deprivation payments	5421	3987
Registration fees	3974	1864
Child health surveillance	5394	1142
Target payments:		
Cervical cytology	8989	7166
Childhood immunizations	6279	6566
Pre-school boosters	2330	1643
	126 624	106 041
Sessional payments		
Health promotion payments	12 236	6032
Minor surgery	5324	4896
Teaching medical students	854	265
	18 414	11 193
Item of service fees		
Night visits	2531	5468
Temporary residents	1453	1215
Contraceptive services	5197	4217
Emergency treatment and INT	115	22
Maternity	8926	7092
Vaccinations and immunizations	4201	4366
	22 423	22 380
Total	211 961	176 925

Figure 11.2 Fees and allowances received by a practice

accounts, the amount of the funds due to the partners. Thus the balance sheet contains:

- assets
- liabilities
- partners' funds.

Accordingly, the net assets of the partnership, which comprise its assets less its liabilities, always equal the partners' funds; thus the two halves of the balance sheet should literally balance. Figure 11.3 shows how the balance sheet distinguishes between partners' funds and the use of these for different purposes. The various subheadings on the balance sheet are described below.

The difference between fixed and current assets

An asset may be defined as something owned by the business and available for its future use.

Fixed assets are those used by the business over a period of several years to help earn profits, but not actually available for resale. These are depreciated to spread their cost over their working life and to apportion the cost (as far as possible) appropriately among the relevant partners.

Conversely, current assets are acquired for sale and conversion into cash during the normal course of the practice's business; for example, dispensing drugs are acquired for resale to generate profit.

The term 'debtors' is used to describe monies owed to the practice for goods or services already provided which are convertible into cash, which is itself a current asset.

The difference between current and long-term liabilities

Current liabilities are amounts owed by the practice and payable within 12 months of the end of the accounting year. These include creditors, amounts due to former partners, capital repayments of a long-term loan due within the next 12 months, and bank overdrafts, which are always repayable on demand!

Long-term liabilities are capital amounts outstanding on loans which are repayable over a period longer than 12 months.

DRS SMITH & PARTNERS
BALANCE SHEET
30 JUNE 1996

	1996		1995	
	£	£	£	£
Partners' funds				
Property capital accounts		106 550		100 813
Capital accounts		20 000		20 000
Current accounts		4090		6211
Taxation provisions		15 819		14 608
		146 459		141 632
Fixed assets		359 363		325 260
Current assets				
Stock of drugs	621		712	
Debtors	32 180		26 956	
Balance at building society	12 271		3479	
Cash at bank and in hand	511		8769	
	45 583		39 916	
Current liabilities				
Bank overdraft	1211		–	
Creditors	13 210		9972	
Due to former partners	597		2638	
GPFC loan	6000		–	
	21 018		12 610	
Net current assets		24 565		27 306
		383 928		352 566
Long-term liabilities				
Mortgage loans		237 469		210 934
Net assets		146 459		141 632

Figure 11.3   Division of partners' funds

The total obtained by subtracting liabilities from assets is the partnership's net assets; this figure represents the net worth of the business and is equal to the partners' funds, being their investment in the practice.

Partners' funds

It helps to understand the nature of their investment in the practice if the partners' funds are divided between long-term investments (which can only be withdrawn when they retire from the practice), and those amounts which reflect the difference between partners' profit shares for the year and their drawings from the practice. The latter represents the money which may be withdrawn from the practice when the accounts are finally agreed.

Thus the partners' funds should be divided into these categories:

- property capital accounts
- capital accounts
- current accounts
- taxation provisions.

The property capital account

This is the partners' net equity in the premises and is the difference between the premises' cost or valuation and any outstanding partnership loans.

If the premises are funded by individual partners' personal loans rather than by a partnership loan, the property capital accounts should show the cost or value of the premises and the partners' borrowing will be shown 'off' balance sheet.

Capital accounts

The partners' capital accounts refer to the funds provided for working capital to enable the practice to run smoothly. The amount of this working capital varies between practices, reflecting the net book value of fixed assets (excluding premises) funded by the partners rather than by partnership loans, and also the value of debtors and creditors to a practice. The capital account therefore funds the purchase of fixed assets and the practice's day-to-day expenditure so that it can run without the risk of incurring an overdraft at times when income may be lower than expenditure.

The capital accounts should be established in the partners' profit sharing ratios to ensure that capital funding is on an equitable basis. A partner's share of this capital will remain in the practice until he or she leaves the partnership.

Current accounts

These reflect the difference between partners' share of the profits for the year less the amounts they have withdrawn, superannuation payments, any sum earmarked for tax and any other personal payments made by the practice on behalf of the individual partners. Figure 11.4 shows the information which should be included to allow each partner to analyse changes in their current account during the year.

Leave advances are included in the current account if these are withdrawn by the partners. They are effectively interest free loans repayable by deduction from the Health Authority's quarterly payments, and they therefore do not affect a practice's profit.

Providing for tax liabilities

Making provision for tax payments is essentially a book-keeping exercise. Within the practice's accounts certain amounts are charged to each partner's current account and credited to a tax provision account in the same partner's name. Payments to the Inland Revenue are drawn from these tax provision accounts. This does not necessarily require the tax to be deposited in a separate bank or building society account; it simply retains the cash in the partnership by preventing partners from withdrawing it from their current accounts. This retained money can be used by the practice as working capital, particularly since it is comparatively easy to plan in advance for its payment to the Inland Revenue.

This arrangement has the advantage of ensuring that each partner's tax liabilities have been provided for. So long as partners' drawings are calculated on a 'net of tax' basis, there should always be enough funds in the tax provision accounts to meet a partner's tax liability.

To illustrate this, the amount of tax provision in accounts for the year ended 30 June 1996 should be sufficient to cover the whole of the 1995/96 liability and any earlier years not yet finally settled, and also one-quarter of the 1996/97 tax liability for the period from 6 April to 30 June 1996.

Figure 11.5 illustrates a partnership taxation provision, and movements within the individual partners' tax provision accounts are shown in Figure 11.6.

Partners' current accounts

	Dr Smith £	Dr Jones £	Dr Green £	Dr Patel £	Total £
Balance at 1 July 1995	1011	2196	1976	1028	6211
Profit for the year	49 304	49 054	44 763	43 067	186 188
Leave advances	1277	1277	1277	1277	5108
Cash introduced	210	–	–	–	210
Income tax repaid	971	1134	56	–	2161
	52 773	53 661	48 072	45 372	199 878
Monthly drawings	29 914	26 699	27 886	28 719	113 218
Fees retained privately	681	315	100	750	1846
Payment of personal expenses	210	–	–	195	405
Spouses' salaries	2521	2422	2456	–	7399
Leave advances withdrawn	1277	1277	1277	1277	5108
Prior shares withdrawn	6525	6662	2025	2025	17 237
Transfers to property capital accounts	1434	1435	1434	1434	5737
Transfers to tax provisions (see Figure 11.5)	5829	6639	7121	5111	24 700
PAYE on appointments	–	1211	519	519	2249
Class 1 NIC	–	283	127	127	537
Class 2 NIC	252	252	252	252	1008
Superannuation:					
Standard	2569	2411	2201	2032	9213
Added years	–	1211	576	–	1787
Appointments	–	572	–	572	1144
Leave advances repaid	1050	1050	1050	1050	4200
	52 262	52 439	47 024	44 063	195 788
Balance at 30 June 1996	511	1222	1048	1309	4090

Figure 11.4   Partners' current accounts

Fundholding and partnership accounts

Fundholders have to produce a separate account for their fundholding activities and these must be drawn up to 31 March each year, regardless of the accounting year of the main practice account. However, there is some interaction between the fundholding and main practice accounts.

The management allowance

This is paid to a practice to cover fundholding management expenses. Thus, in both the preparatory year and the fundholding years, the allowance and its related expenditure must be shown as separate items in the income and expenditure account if it is used to pay for revenue expense items. This ensures that the expenditure is included gross for Review Body purposes.

Reimbursement of capital expenditure, both out of the management allowance and from the savings account, should be shown in the same way as grants in the fixed asset note to the accounts, thus reducing the cost of the assets to the amount contributed by the practice. In most cases this will be nil. However, capital allowances may be claimed on any net amount contributed to the cost of the asset by the practice.

The fundholding bank account

Funds held in this account are not owned by a practice's partners. Therefore the account should be clearly annotated by the bank as a fundholding account, and should not be referred to in the practice balance sheet. Any interest charged on this account should be paid from the management allowance. The partners are not entitled to any interest received on the fundholding account; it must be paid to the Health Authority. Therefore, such interest should not be shown as income in the partnership accounts or in partners' personal tax returns.

Practice staff reimbursement

Reimbursement out of the fundholding staff fund to the partnership must be included in the practice accounts as practice staff refunds, and care should be taken to ensure that all monies due at the year end are included. If too much or too little cash has been transferred from the fundholding bank account, a balance will appear on the fundholding balance sheet as either a debtor or creditor under the heading of general practice account, and an equal and opposite entry should appear in the partnership balance sheet.

Partnership taxation provision

Provision has been made in the accounts for income tax and Class 4 NIC liabilities up to 30 June 1996.

	£
1994/95 estimated repayment due	(1393)
1995/96 balance of liability	14 854
1996/97 on preceding year basis for the period	
6 April 1996–30 June 1996	2358
	15 819

The 1996/97 income tax and Class 4 NIC liabilities (against which £2358 has been provided) are estimated to be:

	£
1996/97 due 1 January 1997	4750
due 1 July 1997	4750
	9500

Figure 11.5 A partnership tax provision

Figure 11.7 shows the note which should appear in the partnership accounts summarizing the expenditure from the fundholding management allowance and the allowance received. It will be seen that the allowance received in respect of revenue items totalled £24 916, and the relevant expenditure is shown in the income and expenditure account in Figure 11.1. The allowance received to reimburse capital acquisitions totalled £8084, and will be set off against the cost of those items in the fixed assets note, thereby reducing the value of the fixed assets on the balance sheet.

Partners' personal expenses

Partners' personal expenses, such as the cost of running cars, can be shown in either the partnership accounts or claimed against tax through their personal tax returns.

Movements on taxation provision

	Dr Smith £	Dr Patel £	Dr Green £	Dr Jones £	Subtotal £	Payments on account £	Total £
Provision brought forward at 1 July 1995	12 124	10 457	13 194	11 122	46 897	(32 289)	14 608
Charge/(release) for:							
1994/95	(1173)	40	(1020)	(5)	(2158)		(2158)
1995/96	6381	6088	7832	4199	24 500		24 500
1996/97	621	511	309	917	2358		2358
Total charge for year	5829	6639	7121	5111	24 700		24 700
(Paid)/repaid during year for:							
1994/95						(11 449)	(11 449)
1995/96						(12 040)	(12 040)
Total payment						(23 489)	(23 489)
Allocation of payment for:							
1993/94	(5013)	(6616)	(6884)	(4738)	(23 251)	23 251	–
Provision carried forward	12 940	10 480	13 431	11 495	48 346	(32 527)	15 819
Representing:							
1994/95	5598	4047	6055	3394	19 094	(20 487)	(1393)
1995/96	6721	5922	7067	7184	26 894	(12 040)	14 854
1996/97	621	511	309	917	2358	–	2358
	12 940	10 480	13 431	11 495	48 346	(32 527)	15 819

Figure 11.6 Movements on partners' tax provision accounts

The Inland Revenue treats the assessable profits for GPs as being the profit as shown in the accounts less the total of the partners' personal expense claims for the same period. Therefore the way in which these expenses are treated does not affect either the timing or the level of tax relief allowed.

Similarly, the Review Body includes partners' personal expense claims in their calculation of total expenses, and again there is no difference between claiming the expenses through the practice accounts or a personal tax return. It is important to note that under self assessment, expenses and capital allowances will only be able to be claimed on the partnership tax return. It will therefore be necessary for partners to disclose their personal expenses and capital allowances to their partners so that they can be incorporated in the personal expenses claim.

The treatment chosen should be that which is most equitable between the partners. If expenses are incurred by all partners at a similar level, they may be included in the partnership accounts without the risk of one partner bearing another's expenses.

However, if there is any element of personal choice which could affect expenses levels, it is much fairer to regard personal expenditure as being paid out of that partner's profit share and tax relief should be claimed on personal expenses claims. Cars are probably the best example of this kind of expenditure; partners usually prefer to buy cars costing significantly different amounts and have widely differing levels of private usage.

The proportion of allowable motoring costs is based on the business usage proportion; thus if a partner is able to claim 80% of usage as business usage, this proportion of motoring costs will be eligible for tax relief. Capital allowances are available on the car irrespective of whether it is owned by the partnership or the partner, and the same rules apply.

Examples of business expenses frequently claimed as personal expenses include:

- surgery facilities in private homes
- home study facilities
- medical books and journals
- courses and conferences
- home telephone bills
- laundry and cleaning
- spouse's salary for telephone answering, secretarial and counselling services.

Fundholding management allowance

		1996 £		1995 £
Allowance received for capital assets		8084		2350
Allowance received for revenue expenditure		24 916		12 646
		33 000		14 996

Capital expenditure				
Computer equipment	6619		–	
Medical equipment	1215		1454	
Furniture and fittings	250		896	
		8084		2350

Revenue expenditure				
Staff salaries	17 456		5432	
Locum payments	2200		2000	
Staff training	2468		1851	
Computer costs and maintenance	1246		563	
Accountancy fees	1546		1176	
Sundry expenses	–		146	
		24 916		11 168
Net income		–		1478

Figure 11.7 Summary of expenditure from the fundholding management allowance

Statistical analysis and review

Accountants with a lengthy and detailed knowledge of medical accounts should be able to 'read' the accounts and identify both areas for concern and areas where the practice has performed well.

Most medical accounting specialists should be able to provide a detailed statistical analysis of the accounts and interpret the results. There are many published statistics relating to GPs and some accountants have additional facilities to provide comparisons with regional data. Perhaps the most important statistics are those which provide an analysis of NHS income. Statistics for gross NHS income, net NHS income, item of service fees and the allocation of NHS fees should be considered as a minimum. These provide good overall indicators of the practice's performance for the year when compared to national, regional and prior year's figures.

A review of the accounts is also helpful in enabling the partners to interpret the accounts and highlight good and bad areas of the practice finances. The review should cover: incoming and outgoing partners, profit sharing arrangements, an interpretation of profit variances from previous years, a review of income and expenditure, partners' capital, and any other matters of relevance to the current or succeeding accounting period.

Partnership deed

It is important that the current, valid and signed partnership agreement be provided to the accountant with the practice's accounting records. This enables the accountant to ensure that current practice policies are reflected in the accounts.

Where a partnership agreement does not exist, the accountant is likely to ask for a letter of representation to be signed by the partners. This is a letter which sets out many basic common practices regarding profit sharing arrangements etc. The letter of representation should not be used and is not intended for use as a permanent replacement for a partnership deed.

12 Taxation

For young doctors entering general practice, the strange and arcane world of GP finance can be something of a culture shock to those more familiar with the relatively simple methods of tax and National Insurance deduction at source. Having come to terms with the payment of tax under Schedule D, the various classes of National Insurance and the like represents a major change and fortunate is the young GP with an advisor who is prepared to explain this to him; to help him through the period of change and to ensure that nothing works to his financial disadvantage.

This chapter looks at the manner in which GPs' profits are taxed under the regulations applying to all self-employed taxpayers, whether in partnership or sole practice. This chapter does not aim to set out full details of the UK tax system as it applies to GPs; and readers requiring further clarification should seek expert advice or refer to further available publications.

Taxation of some kind has, like the poor, always been with us and presumably will remain so. It comes in several forms; taxes on income, on capital, on the estates of deceased persons, value added tax levied on goods and services, to name but a few. The average GP is likely to come across most, if not all, of these forms of taxation during his working life.

The regulation of all our taxes is based upon Acts of Parliament passed from time to time which lay down, in general terms, the means by which those taxes will be levied and how they will be administered and collected. Each November the Chancellor of the Exchequer presents to Parliament a Budget Statement, which ultimately finds its way on to the statute book as the latest Finance Act for that year.

The Inland Revenue offices: inspection and collection

Broadly speaking, the revenue service so far as the GP is concerned, is divided into two sections; the Inspector and Collector. It is the Inspector of Taxes office with whom an accountant will negotiate in order to agree his client's tax liability. The office will be staffed by revenue officials of various grades who will each have their separate function to perform. It is that office which will issue assessment notices, to which appeals will be sent and correspondence conducted.

The Collector of Taxes offices throughout the country, on the other hand, are responsible purely for the demand and collection of tax. It is they to whom a tax bill will be paid, who will deal with the issue of receipts and take enforcement proceedings if the tax is not paid. At times, the liaison between the two offices may not be as efficient as it should be!

The Schedules

Income tax is divided into a number of schedules, each of which governs the rules for assessment of tax on incomes of various types. For most GPs, Schedules D and E are of relevance and we shall look at these in some detail.

Employment and self-employment: Schedules D and E

For most GPs it will be the tax upon their incomes which will concern them the most and in which only Schedules D and E will be concerned.

Most GPs at some time will have been assessed for tax under Schedule E and have had deductions made from their salaries under PAYE. They will have, at various times, been employees of a hospital authority; GP trainees or in other forms of employment. The GP, on the other hand, as a self-employed practitioner is assessed under Schedule D, which in itself derives entirely from his status as an independent contractor.

As the method of assessment in each case is entirely different, it is important to understand how these schedules work. The main differences lie in the manner in which expenses are allowed; the basis of assessment; dates of payment of tax. These rules apply to all self-employed taxpayers, not merely GPs. To make matters perhaps even more confusing, in many cases these two schedules overlap, with doctors receiving income simultaneously under both headings. Where this occurs in partnerships, extremely complex situations can arise. In many cases too, it is not immediately apparent whether the income from any particular appointment is to be assessed under Schedule D or Schedule E. In recent years, the Inland Revenue has looked at a number of professions, quite outside the medical world, and these have been re-designated from Schedule E to Schedule D. The benefits to the Revenue are obvious.

In the medical field, such confusion can frequently arise in the treatment of fees paid to locums or assistant doctors. Where fees are paid from practice funds to such a doctor, extreme care must be taken to ensure that the proper taxation formalities are observed. If, for instance, a practice engages a doctor at a salary of £15 000 a year and then proceeds to pay that doctor monthly, this is in every sense of the word a salary and must be taxed under PAYE. If, on the other hand, occasional locum fees are paid to different doctors, calculated on a sessional basis without any true employer/employee relationship, then it is likely that they can be treated as Schedule D income in the hands of the recipient, who will himself bear the obligation of returning these to the Inland Revenue and paying tax on them.

Years of assessment

For everyone in the country, doctors or not, tax is organized on the basis of tax years, sometimes termed 'years of assessment' or 'fiscal years'. In all cases, and however assessed, these years run from 6 April in one calendar year to 5 April in the next. Thus, the year from 6 April 1994 to 5 April 1995 would be designated 1994/95, and that from 6 April 1995 to 5 April 1996 as 1995/96.

The preceding year (PY) basis

Up to 1995/96, all GPs were taxed on the PY basis, which means that for any one fiscal year the profits taxed in that year will be those generated in the accounting period ended in the previous fiscal year. Therefore, for a practice making up its accounts to, say, 30 June 1993, the profits will have been taxed in the fiscal year 1994/95.

The preceding year basis has now effectively ended. During the change to current year basis the last year to which this applied was 1995/96, so that in the example given, profits for that year would be taxed on the basis of those earned in the year to 30 June 1994.

The preceding year basis is now passing into history and will not be further considered in this chapter.

The current year (CY) basis of assessment

With the ending of the PY basis, a new system of taxing the self-employed will be introduced, the CY basis, whereby profits will be taxed on the basis of the account period ended *within* (rather than previous to) the year of assessment. Thus, using the same example, profits earned in the year to 30 June 1998 will be taxed in the year 1998/99.

By this means, those profits earned for any given year will be taxed 12 months earlier than would formerly have been the case. Figure 12.1 shows the manner in which these profits will be taxed and the years on which assessments will be raised.

The transitional year

As will be seen, the last year to which the PY basis applies will be 1995/96, whilst the first full year to which the CY basis applies will be 1997/98. It will be seen that there are two accounting years missing and one tax year, 1996/97. The Revenue has decided therefore that profits for the year 1996/97, known as the transitional year, will be based upon the average of those earned within the two accounting periods concerned. On that basis the total of £380 000 earned in the two years up to 30 June 1996 will be halved and the average of £190 000 will represent the taxable profits for 1996/97.

ACCOUNTS YEAR ENDED 30 JUNE

Year to 30 June	Profit £	Taxed in Year		Profits Taxed £
1993	150 000	1994/95	(PY)	150 000
1994	170 000	1995/96	(PY)	170 000
1995	180 000 }	1996/97	(T)	190 000
1996	200 000			
1997	220 000	1997/98	(CY)	220 000
1998	225 000	1998/99	(CY)	225 000
1999	245 000	1999/2000	(CY)	245 000

PY: Preceding year basis
CY: Current year basis
T: Transitional year

Figure 12.1   The change to current year basis

Partnerships

The vast majority of GPs practise as members of groups or partnerships, the main characteristic of which is that they share profits in some pre-arranged ratios. At the last count, of some 33 000 GPs practising in the UK about 81% were working as members of partnerships. Almost certainly the new doctor will find this first experience of general practice as a principal, or junior partner, working his way to parity over an agreed period.

The tax rules for the computation of profits assessable on partnerships and individual partners are complex, and are likely to remain so. Up to 1996/97, profits have been assessed on the partnership and demands for tax issued in the partnership name. These have invariably been apportioned by the practice accountant in accordance with the personal reliefs and expenses allowed in respect of each individual partner. The actual amount of tax payable by the partnership was therefore the sum total of the individual partner's own tax liabilities. These can vary widely, even between equal members of the same partnership.

With the advent of self-assessment these composite partnership assessments will no longer be issued. In their place, partnership tax returns will have to be submitted to the Revenue which sets out in precise terms the amount of assessable profits attributable to each individual partner. Those will then be transferred to the partners' own individual tax returns and tax paid according to the rules of self assessment.

Joint and several liability

Up to 5 April 1997, partners were jointly and severally liable for the tax liability of their partnership. Thus, if one partner defaulted or could not be found when the tax fell due for settlement, the onus for payment could well fall back on his own (or former) partners. So far as the Inland Revenue was involved, it was no concern of theirs from whom the tax originated, so long as their demands were settled.

This was a prospect which most partnerships were only too anxious to avoid. This was, in many cases, dealt with by partnerships setting funds aside, either in a building society or bank deposit account, so that they were available when settlement was due.

This concept of joint and several liability has now effectively ceased, from the 1997/98 tax year, although it will in effect continue in a diminishing manner and will apply to all tax years where tax has not been settled up to and including 1996/97. From 6 April 1997, liabilities will be chargeable only to individual partners through their personal tax returns and no liability will fall on the partnership or other partners.

Income tax reserves

Those partnerships who have habitually, and as a matter of policy, set aside funds to meet these tax liabilities should now consider carefully whether they wish to do so, in the light of the ending of joint and several liability.

Experience shows that many such partnerships wish to continue to reserve funds in this manner, in order to even out their cash flow and to ensure that separate partners are not required to draw substantial cheques at six monthly intervals. This is a policy matter which, with sound professional advice, should be considered by each individual partnership.

Self assessment

Up to the 1995/96 year, most doctors would receive a tax return which they were committed to completing and returning to the Inland Revenue. The only sanction available to the Revenue was that if the return was not submitted by 31 October in each year and there were any undeclared sources of income or capital gains tax upon which tax was due, interest would then be charged. All this has changed; a much more draconian regime has been introduced with heavy penalties applying where tax-payers do not submit the return within specified time limits.

These self assessment procedures involve the completion of annual tax returns which are much more complex than those previously issued and which in themselves provide for settlement of the tax due by the taxpayer. Originally introduced by the Revenue as 'simplification' of income tax, it appears likely to be nothing of the sort and for a high proportion of doctors who for some reason find it impossible to submit their returns on time, it will almost certainly result in heavy penalties being charged.

It has been estimated that self assessment procedures will apply to some nine million taxpayers. Estimates of those who will be involved in the penalty regime have varied from one to three million.

Issue and submission of returns

Self assessment returns will be issued to those who generally completed tax returns previously – to all self-employed people, partners, those liable to higher rate tax, with unearned and investment income etc. Returns will be issued by the Revenue around 6 April each year.

The returns themselves, with numerous supporting schedules, will be very different from the old style tax returns, requiring the completion of boxes and calculation of tax payable. Where it is intended that the Revenue will calculate the tax payable, the return must be submitted to the tax office by 30 September after the fiscal year concerned. Thus, for the 1997/98 year a return for that purpose must be submitted by 30 September 1998. Where the taxpayer proposes to calculate his own tax liability, then the return must be submitted to the Revenue by 31 January of the following year. Failure to submit the return by the latter of these two dates will result in an immediate penalty of £100, escalating substantially where this delay is prolonged for any length of time.

Record keeping under self assessment

There are, for the first time, guidelines set down by the Inland Revenue for the keeping of records both by personal taxpayers and those in business, such as GPs. These regulations require businesses to keep full records of their business transactions, which include details of receipts and payments, cash expenses etc. In an extreme case where records are produced and are quite clearly inadequate, the Revenue is empowered to levy penalties up to £3000.

Dates of payment of tax

Many GPs will have been used to paying tax on 1 January and 1 July each year under self assessment. This system continued until 1995/96 for those in sole practice, and they will now pay tax from 1996/97 on 31 January and 31 July each year. For partnerships, the system has remained in place for 1996/97 but they will commence the new payment dates from 1997/98.

Tax payable will consist of a first and second instalment payable on those dates each year, together with a balancing-up from the previous year on the following 31 January. Thus, where a practice is to pay tax on 31 January 1998, this payment will consist of the first instalment of the tax for 1997/98, together with a balancing payment from 1996/97.

Hospital remuneration in partnerships

In many partnerships, doctors receive part of the practice remuneration in the form of 'salaries', frequently for clinical assistant posts at local hospitals. Where this applies, the income will be included in the partnership accounts, invariably because of a policy of aggregation of profits from medical sources by the partnership. A clause of this type may well be included in the partnership deed.

The system by which this income is taxed is complex. Until recently, a major difficulty was caused by local tax offices insisting on taxing this upon the recipient even though it was not legally his own money. This system has now been alleviated and tax offices will issue authority for income of this type to be paid without the deduction of tax. Negotiations to ensure this takes place should be conducted through the practice accountant.

The property owning partnership

Surgery premises are invariably held in partnerships and these shares of ownership will frequently differ from those in which practice profits are shared. It is necessary in such circumstances to include transactions applying to the surgery ownership within the normal Schedule D assessment, but dividing the net profit or loss accruing in the shares in which the building is owned during the year of assessment. The surgery premises should always be included in the practice balance sheet, whether or not it is owned by all the partners.

Personal practice expenses

There are few areas which cause such controversy in the world of GP finance as the extent and manner in which the doctor is to claim tax relief in respect of expenses paid privately, but which involve wholly or partly an element of practice use. It is an area which is likely to bring the GP into conflict with his accountant and, possibly through him, with the Inland Revenue.

As we shall see, the attitude of the Inland Revenue has hardened considerably in recent years and, if detected, the over-claiming of these expenses by GPs can cost the doctor dearly. What we are talking about, as likely as not, are expenses which fall under a number of headings but which are likely to be paid by the doctor personally rather than through his partnership. Each partner will submit, or have prepared for him by his accountant, an annual claim for personal practice expenses which is allowable against tax in exactly the same manner as partnership profits are assessed, i.e. on the current year basis. Therefore, if five doctors are in a partnership making up its annual accounts to 30 June, each of them will prepare a practice expenses claim made up to 30 June annually. Doctors are not employees and should not prepare expenses claims up to a 5 April year end unless this happens to coincide with the annual accounting date of the partnership.

These expenses, once formulated and agreed with the Inland Revenue, will be allowed for tax against that partner's share of the profits and no other. In large partnerships one can find that these expenses claims for partners vary widely, normally for perfectly good reasons; there is no reason whatever why partners will have the same personal circumstances and it is quite common for there to be large differences in the amounts each partner will claim. This will inevitably have an effect on their own share of the partnership tax liability.

Partnership and personal expenses

For the vast majority of expenditure met by the doctor or, more likely, his partnership, there is no argument whatever and the Inland Revenue is highly unlikely to dispute expenditure on such routine and non-controversial expenses as printing and stationery, surgery telephone bills, staff wages, locum fees etc.

The categories of expenditure paid personally will vary between one partnership and another. It is up to the partners themselves to determine exactly what expenditure is paid out of partnership funds and what is paid privately by the partners. Whatever they decide, however, should be mutually agreed between them and ideally should be set out clearly in the partnership deed. It is important for an incoming partner to check exactly what expenses he will be asked to bear personally. To preserve fairness, the same rule should apply to all partners regardless of their status in the partnership.

The basic rule

The basic rule applicable to the claiming of these expenses, for Schedule D purposes, is that they must be seen by the Inland Revenue as having been expended wholly and exclusively for the purpose of the profession. Thus, the GP who pays locum fees to another doctor for covering him in out-of-hours duties, will without question get those fees allowed for income tax. If he were an employed doctor, it is highly unlikely that he would get them allowed because the additional qualifying word, 'necessarily', might be impossible to justify.

Claims for personal practice expenses in respect of doctors in partnership should always be made up to the same date as the practice's accounting year end, even though a doctor joined mid-way through the year. Thus, if Dr E joined his partnership on 1 February 1997 and the partnership makes up its accounts to 30 June annually, his first claim should be for the five month period to 30 June 1997 and to the same annual date in succeeding years.

Of far greater difficulty are those expenses which the doctor pays out partially for both private and for practice use. Nobody, for instance, will dispute the fact that a doctor needs to use his car or his private telephone for practice purposes; how much exactly in fractional terms that should be is another matter and in the last analysis may be the subject of negotiations between the accountant and the Inland Revenue.

A further doctrine the Inland Revenue may seek to impose is that of 'duality of purpose'. This means that if the expenditure is incurred simultaneously both for private and practice use, the expenditure will be wholly disallowable. This is subject to a number of variations, most of which the average taxpayer may well, with some justification, consider to be 'splitting hairs'. Thus, a doctor who buys his suits to use in his consulting room would be unable to obtain any tax relief for that expenditure. The Revenue considers this to be primarily for a private purpose with some incidental element of practice use. On the other hand, the same principle is unlikely to be applied to such expenses as motor cars. The Inland Revenue fully accepts that there is an element of practice use which is quite clearly allowable. By the same token there will be an element of private use which must be disallowed.

The Inland Revenue attitude

It is fair to say that, historically, GPs have received generous treatment from the Inland Revenue in the scrutiny of their expenses claims. However, there is some clear evidence of a change in approach in more recent years.

As part of a general hardening of attitude to self-employed taxpayers, expenses claims in general are subject to much greater scrutiny than has always been the case in the past. For self-employed GPs, both medical and dental, there is some evidence that their accounts and claims have been subject to a particularly close watch and that Inspectors of Taxes have queried such claims under a number of headings. It seems unlikely that this process will ease with the advent of self assessment.

Experience does tend to show that salaries paid to wives/spouses, motor expenses, practice use of houses and telephone costs are particularly vulnerable. The inclusion of estimates is also attacked in some cases.

Where the Revenue is able to establish a pattern of over-claiming lasting for several years, it is empowered to increase assessments retrospectively, possibly over as much as six years, seeking to collect not only lost tax but interest and penalties too. It is essential that doctors understand that the risk of unrealistic claims sparking off an in-depth investigation is increasing. In particular, it should be ensured that:

- all claims submitted are clearly justified and the expenditure has actually been expended for practice purposes
- receipts are available to support all claims, and
- where restrictions for private use are in force, they can be justified.

Claims showing estimated expenditure are avoided so far as is possible. Where these are unavoidable, the fact that they are estimates should be clearly shown on claims submitted to the Revenue.

GPs should understand that when a claim is prepared on their behalf by an accountant, the onus is upon them not only to keep the accountant informed of genuine expenses incurred but also to check draft claims before submission to ensure that no unjustified or incorrect claims are made. A GP should be asked to sign the claim as correct before it is submitted to the Inland Revenue.

What can be claimed?

Before we go on to look at the various types of claim which might be made, these can fall in a number of generalized categories:

- Expenditure paid personally by the doctor but which can quite clearly be demonstrated as being solely for practice purposes, such as medical equipment, medical journals, subscriptions etc.
- Such expenses as are partially practice and partially private use, such as home telephone, motor cars, etc.
- Expenses which the doctor wishes to claim but can produce no hard and fast evidence and where estimates may be submitted. As outlined above, claims of this nature are particularly at risk of attracting unwanted Revenue attention.

Doctors frequently ask 'What claims am I entitled to make?'. The short answer is that he has no absolute entitlement to claim anything at all. He can look for ever at the Income Tax Acts and find no reference to doctors' cars, houses and the like. Indeed he may claim whatever he wishes but, as has been pointed out, claiming it and having it allowed by the Revenue are two entirely separate matters. The days of over-claiming expenditure and hoping that the Inland Revenue would allow it through 'on the nod' are gone; the penalties for over-claiming make it perfectly clear that the game is not worth the candle.

The preparation of claims of this nature can cause controversy between the GP and his accountant. Let it be clearly understood therefore that the accountant who advises his client to moderate his claims to a level which will be acceptable to the Revenue, yet which at the same time does not deprive the doctor of any tax relief to which he might legitimately be due, is doing no more than attempting to protect his client in advance from the excesses of an Inland Revenue enquiry. He is acting with the long-term interests of his client at heart and the GP should accept and be grateful for advice of this nature.

Who should submit the claim?

In the rare case of a doctor who does not engage an accountant to act for him that GP will submit and formulate his claim himself, agreeing this with the Inland Revenue. Whether this is a process in the best interests of the GP is another matter; he has no specialist knowledge in dealing with the local Inspector of Taxes and this may well be better left to a professional accountant who is an expert at negotiations of this nature.

If the doctor is in sole practice the claim would normally be produced as part of his practice accounts without the necessity for submitting separate claims and no undue difficulty would arise here. It is in the case of doctors in partnerships where problems can arise as to exactly by whom the claim is to be prepared.

At times one comes across instances in partnerships where the doctors chose to have separate accountants to deal with their personal affairs. This is their own prerogative and nobody would seek to take this from them. However, it should be accepted that the accountant who deals with the partnership may well have a superior knowledge of the negotiations which have been conducted with the Inspector of Taxes and there are excellent reasons why, again, the same accountant should act for all the partners in submitting these claims. It may be that he is able to obtain some sort of omnibus agreement from the Inland Revenue, very much to the partners' own advantage. Only if he is acting for all the partners in a practice can they best be able to take advantage of this.

The submission of claims by separate accountants may be done on entirely different bases and if only one of these claims provokes an enquiry from the Inland Revenue, this could spread to all the doctors in the partnership.

Practice use of home

The vast majority of doctors in general practice will use their home to a greater or lesser degree for practice purposes. Some, with no other central surgery, or sole practitioners whose only surgery is in part of their house, will have a perfectly legitimate claim for a major share of the costs of running the house. At the other end of the scale one will come across the GP, probably living several miles away from the practice area who uses his house mainly for occasional study or reference purposes. The claims which these two doctors can justify will in practice be extremely different.

Proportion of house expenses

Claims are frequently made for practice use of doctors' houses, based upon the proportion which the practice use of the house bears to the total floor area or by some similar means. Such claims, possibly when extended to include qualifying repairs expenditure and by excess mortgage interest, can at times be very substantial.

In order to ensure that such claims are justified and in an effort to avoid constant Revenue enquiries, it is generally considered that claims of this nature can only be justified when:

(i) There is clear evidence of the use of the house for consulting or treatment of patients on a regular basis

(ii) A professional plate is displayed outside the house. Though not mandatory, this could make the acceptance of a borderline claim more likely

(iii) There is an appropriate entry in the local telephone directory

(iv) The house is either within, or adjacent to, the practice area

(v) If the claim is to be fully justified, point (i) above must apply.

Having established that the basis for such a claim exists, it is necessary then to go on and calculate the fractional cost of the total house expenses to be claimed. The method usually employed and which is invariably acceptable to the Inland Revenue, is to award an arbitrary points figure to every room in the house, more or less dependent upon its size and then to allocate those points between practice and private use. The system will at times be adapted to a system based upon floor areas; but this may be felt an over-complication and may well give rise to an identical result.

For instance, if there is a study where patients are seen and which is used for no other purpose, the whole of the points attributable to this room can be allocated to practice use. Conversely it is unlikely that an upstairs bedroom or bathroom can be allocated other than wholly for private use. The actual expenses to be included in the claim will be the normal running costs of the house, but excluding capital expenditure.

Study allowance

Where the house is not regularly used for consultations but the doctor, nevertheless, spends time working at home, it is much less contentious to claim a 'study allowance', based on a lump sum estimate of the additional cost to the doctor of using his house for that purpose. A typical annual claim might be:

£1.50 per hour for ten hours per week over 50 weeks a year = £750.

Alternatively, a round sum per week could be claimed.

Capital gains tax

One reason which frequently deters GPs from making a claim for house expenses is that they have been advised, probably incorrectly, that, in the event of the house being sold at a profit at some time in the future, they will be liable for capital gains tax on a proportion of a gain realized. This is, in fact, not the case. In such circumstances CGT would not be charged unless there was some part of the house which was used exclusively for practice purposes. Even if this were the case and the doctor acquired a replacement house, also to be used in his practice, it is likely that the 'roll-over' relief could be claimed.

Although by no means impossible, experience does show that it is highly unlikely that a GP selling a house which has been partially used in his practice will give rise to an actual charge upon which CGT is payable.

The whole subject of CGT on GPs' houses is extremely complex and specialist professional advice should always be sought in such an instance. Suffice to say here that no doctor should be dissuaded from making a legitimate claim for house expenses merely by the prospect, however remote, of having to pay CGT at some time in the future.

Some other claims may include the following:

- **Medical subscriptions:** All GPs pay their registration fee to the GMC and will also subscribe to one of the medical protection societies. They may also be members of the BMA, RCGP and several other societies of a more specific nature within the profession. Care should be taken to see that all these subscriptions are properly recorded and claimed.

- **Charitable and other donations:** Some GPs will make donations to local charities and, provided these are of a reasonable amount, the local Inspector of Taxes will allow them against profits and these again should be properly recorded.

- **Medical books and journals:** Although many GPs receive most literature free of charge, there are still those who subscribe regularly to medical journals, as well as purchasing books.

- **Locum fees etc:** Many GPs make payments to locums for temporarily looking after their practice, as well as payments for deputizing and relief services. In many cases, depending largely on clauses in the partnership deed, these may be made personally by the partners rather than out of partnership funds.

- **Security expenses:** With many doctors keeping valuable drugs and equipment in their houses, the necessity for expenditure on some form of security is obvious. The installation of burglar alarms, annual maintenance of these, provision of security locks, etc should all be claimed for tax purposes.

- **Bank charges:** GPs often use their own private bank account to some degree for practice purposes, e.g. by paying part of their house costs, motor expenses and other sundry items from their private account. If a charge is made by the bank for use of this account, a proportion of the charges (but not interest) can be included in the claim.

- **Cleaning and laundry:** Here again, most of this expense is likely to be paid from the partnership but if privately paid the laundry of overalls, protective clothing etc should be claimed. Claims for the cleaning of normal wear, such as suits and dresses, is unlikely to be accepted unless a particularly good case can be made. Claims for the purchase of such ordinary items of clothing will not be allowed under any circumstances.

- **Medical instruments:** The upkeep of cleaning and replacing medical equipment is again a perfectly proper claim and all amounts should be carefully listed and included under this heading.

- **Waiting room papers and flowers:** Here again, this is often included in overall house expenses and reduced accordingly. It is preferable to claim this as a separate entity if justified.

- **Accountancy fees:** Most of the practice accountancy bills will be paid from partnership funds but if any charges are made to individual doctors for personal expenses claims etc these should be claimed. No claim can be made, however the bill is paid, for dealing with a doctor's personal income tax return.

- **Insurance premiums:** The insurance on the house will normally be included in a house expenses claim. Motor insurance should be included in the claim for car expenses. There are, however, a few premiums which can be included under general practice expenses; public liability insurance and medical surgical equipment. Life assurance payments do not qualify for relief.

- **'Locum insurance' payments:** For many years it was accepted that where doctors paid into policies which provided a benefit in the event of sickness or accident, there was no tax relief on those premiums. This ruling has now changed, with an announcement by the Inland Revenue during 1996 that where those premiums were paid on genuine locum insurance policies, i.e. those which provide for a repayment of locum costs incurred, then the premiums on those policies will be allowable for tax purposes. In the event of a benefit being paid under the policy, any amount received would then rank as chargeable income in the hands of the recipient.

It must be emphasized that the majority of these policies are written as permanent health insurance policies, which provide for the payment of a lump sum in the event of absence through sickness or injury, whether or not locums are engaged. These premiums will continue to be disallowed for tax purposes, although any benefit will continue to be not chargeable to tax.

- **Courses, conferences etc:** In many cases, costs of attending courses are refunded from NHS sources and, where no net cost is met by the GP, obviously no claim can be made. However, there are other conferences which can be attended at the GP's own cost and a claim must be made for these. Difficulty may be experienced in having claims for major overseas conferences accepted. If accompanied by a spouse, the Inspector of Taxes is likely to insist that his or her share of the costs is excluded from the claim.

- **Private telephone bills:** In some partnerships, it is the policy of the practice that all private telephone accounts are paid from partnership funds. However, in other cases, these will be met personally and a proportion of the cost of the calls should be included in the claim. This will be a matter of record and negotiation. Some Inspectors of Taxes will also allow a proportion of the rental charge. VAT is included on private telephone bills and this should also be included.

- **Photographic expenses:** Many GPs use cameras for genuine medical reasons, often in connection with training purposes. This is a perfectly reasonable claim to make, although here again some element of private use may have to be taken into account.

- **Maintenance of approach:** The cost of maintaining the garden and surroundings of the house used by the practice can be claimed in several ways. The actual cost of the upkeep of the approach to the house, to the extent that this is likely to be used by patients, is a proper claim either by inclusion in an overall claim for house expenses or separately.

- **Computers and technical equipment:** The use by GPs of personally owned computers, video equipment etc is increasing. Where such equipment is bought and retained in the doctor's private house, some difficulty may be experienced in having the claim agreed as the Revenue is aware that this is likely to be used to a large degree for private and recreational purposes. If, however, such equipment were bought by the practice, included as a partnership asset and retained in the surgery, little difficulty is likely to be encountered.

National Insurance

The young GP will find that National Insurance is no longer deducted from his salary. These Class 1 contributions, paid by employees only, are deducted automatically and are calculated by the employer. There is no action the employed doctor need take. As a GP, he will be liable to pay NIC under Class 2 and Class 4. Class 2 contributions are a weekly payment (for 1997/98: £6.15). These are normally paid either by direct debit to a bank account or by settling a monthly bill issued by the DSS.

The young doctor joining a practice must be extremely careful to ensure that he registers as self-employed and pays these contributions as and when they fall due. Failure to do so could well result in a large bill submitted at some time in the future.

Class 4 contributions are paid with the annual tax demand and are currently levied at 6% on a band of profits. For 1997/98, the maximum amount payable by GPs is £1030 p.a.

BMA Professional Services Ltd (BMAPS)

BMAPS was set up in early 1996 to offer accountancy, financial and taxation advice to BMA members. The company is wholly owned by the BMA and acts only for BMA members.

BMAPS operates as a conventional accounting firm, except that profits generated are ploughed back into the BMA for the benefit of members. Fees are charged on the basis of an agreed sum at the start of the year which will not normally be revised. This allows doctors to budget their personal outgoings much more effectively than would otherwise be the case. BMAPS is staffed by accountants experienced in working for doctors.

Over the next three years, BMAPS will be expanding nationwide. It currently has offices in the following areas: South Thames based in Caterham (Tel: 01883 331215); North Thames based in Wembley (Tel: 0181 900 0444); and Trent based in Nottingham (Tel: 0115 948 0788). Any enquiries can be directed to BMAPS at BMA House (Tel: 0171 383 6743).

The Association of Independent Specialist Medical Accounts (AISMA)

For general practices in areas not covered by the BMAPS service, GPs seeking the services of an accredited specialist accountant might like to contact AISMA, an association of local accounting firms who have been accepted as members of the Association. This is the only such organization in the country catering for accountants specializing in work for GPs. The telephone number is 01424 730345.

13 Superannuation

Many GPs only take an interest in their pensions just before they retire. Though understandable, this may be unfortunate because at this late stage the opportunities to change pension arrangements are very limited. Ideally, everyone should be familiar with their pension arrangements and keep them under review.

The NHS pension scheme (NHSPS)

The NHSPS has two distinct benefit structures: one for independent contractors (mainly GPs) and one for salaried employees (including hospital doctors). Salaried employees are pensioned on a traditional final salary/

years of service basis. GPs on the other hand are pensioned using a unique method which takes into account all superannuable income earned throughout their careers. This method was specifically designed for GPs so as to take account of their career pattern, i.e. earnings tend to peak earlier and may even decline as they approach retirement.

Membership of the NHSPS

Membership of the scheme is open to principal practitioners, associates and assistants approved by Health Authorities. Most non-principals, including locums, retainer scheme doctors and non-approved assistants are not able to join the scheme (except locums appointed by a Health Authority). However, the scheme is to be opened to GP practice staff from 1 September 1997 and the BMA will press for non-principals to be permitted to join as well. GP registrars and salaried GPs are eligible to join but are pensioned using the salaried employee method rather than the special GP method.

Superannuable income

For pension purposes, GP income is divided into three groups, as set out in Box 13.1 below.

Box 13.1: The NHS pension scheme – superannuable income

Group 1: payments which are not superannuable.

These consist entirely of the reimbursement of expenses for superannuation purposes:

- all payments, except the trainers' grant, made in respect of a GP registrar. (Payments of salary and board and lodging should be treated as the superannuable income of the registrar)
- payments and notional reimbursements under the schemes for rent and rates and practice staff
- payments in respect of the employment of a locum under the schemes for additional payments during sickness and confinement and payments for prolonged study leave
- payments under the doctors' retainer scheme

continued opposite

Box 13.1: *continued*

- associate allowance
- direct payments for computing costs
- locum payments for single-handed rural GPs attending training courses
- payments made in accordance with LIZ Workforce Flexibilities
  - Type 3 IPA
  - LIZ collaborative working allowance
  - LIZ associate doctor payment
  - LIZ assistants scheme
- payments under the out-of-hours development scheme.

Group 2: payments which are fully superannuable.

These consist entirely of net income for superannuation purposes:

- additions to basic practice allowance (BPA) for practice in a designated area
- addition to BPA for seniority
- a training grant under the trainee practitioner scheme
- inducement payments
- transitional payments (1990–91/1991–92 scheme)
- target payments for childhood immunization, pre-school boosters and cervical cytology.

Group 3: payments which are partly superannuable.

These consist partly of reimbursement of expenses and partly of net income for superannuation purposes. The expenses element is reviewed regularly and is currently 30.9%, so that 69.1% is superannuable:

- dispensing fees, on-cost and oxygen therapy service rents and fees paid in respect of the supply of drugs and appliances
- basic practice allowance (BPA)

continued overleaf

Box 13.1: *continued*

- additions to BPA for the employment of an assistant; *including* the higher allowance when a principal is also receiving an addition to BPA for practice in a designated area but *excluding* payments under the LIZ assistants scheme
- standard capitation fees
- fees for vaccination and immunization carried out for reasons of public policy
- night visit fees
- contraceptive service fees
- maternity medical service fees
- payments for treating temporary residents and providing immediately necessary treatment
- fees for providing treatment in an emergency, for the arrest of dental haemorrhage and where a second practitioner is required to administer an anaesthetic
- initial practice allowance Types 1 and 2 only; Type 3 payments to GPs in LIZ area are non-superannuable
- rural practice payments
- postgraduate education allowance
- minor surgery sessional fees
- payment for health promotion programmes and chronic disease management programmes (including payments made under transitional arrangements)
- child health surveillance fees
- deprivation fees (including payments made under transitional arrangements)
- registration fees
- fees for involvement in undergraduate medical education
- capitation additions for out-of-hours cover.

Contributions

GPs contribute 6% of their superannuable income. Although self-employed and therefore not statutorily entitled to tax relief, GPs do receive tax relief as a result of a special extra-statutory concession.

Superannuable practice income will be divided amongst the partners by the Health Authority/Board according to their profit-sharing ratios. The Health Authority/Board will provide an annual statement (form SD86C) to GPs showing the superannuable income credited to them during the year ending 31 March. This information needs to be checked carefully on receipt.

Dynamizing

Because all NHS superannuable income earned throughout a career is taken into account in calculating a GP's pension, it is essential that this income is protected against inflation over the years. This protection is provided by the procedure known as dynamizing. This involves the GP's superannuable income being uprated by a factor which reflects the annual review body award. Dynamized income for every year of the GP's career is added together and this total figure is used to calculate the pension (see below). The current uprating factor this year is shown in Box 13.2.

Pension

A GP's pension is calculated by multiplying total dynamized income by 1.4%. For example, a doctor who has worked for 37 years as a GP and accumulated total dynamized income of £1 517 000:

$$\text{Pension is:} \quad £1\ 517\ 000 \times 1.4\% = £21\ 238.$$

The pension is increased in line with the retail prices index each year.

Lump sum

In addition, there is a tax free lump sum of three times the pension. In the above example, the lump sum would be:

$$£21\ 238 \times 3 = £63\ 714$$

Box 13.2: Uprating (dynamizing) factors applied to GPs' superannuable pay to calculate pension

Year ending 31 March	Uprating factor	Year ending 31 March	Uprating factor
1949	26.684	1974	7.736
1950	26.684	1975	7.077
1951	24.685	1976	5.093
1952	24.685	1977	4.963
1953	24.685	1978	4.776
1954	24.685	1979	3.662
1955	24.685	1980	3.114
1956	24.685	1981	2.624
1957	24.563	1982	2.475
1958	22.297	1983	2.342
1959	21.989	1984	2.193
1960	21.022	1985	2.058
1961	20.101	1986	1.916
1962	20.101	1987	1.803
1963	20.101	1988	1.657
1964	17.631	1989	1.545
1965	17.631	1990	1.430
1966	16.030	1991	1.323
1967	14.897	1992	1.186
1968	12.022	1993	1.112
1969	11.784	1994	1.095
1970	11.121	1995	1.062
1971	9.267	1996	1.031
1972	8.579	1997	1.000
1973	7.979		

However, for married men, service before 1972 only attracts lump sum at one times the pension, not three times. They will therefore have a lump sum less than three times pension unless they paid extra contributions in order to purchase the full unreduced lump sum (see below).

Other scheme benefits

These include:

- a widow's pension of 50% of the doctor's pension. For a female doctor, the widower's pension is 50% of the doctor's pension earned since 1988 only
- children's allowance if a GP dies and has children under the age of 17 or in full-time education
- tax free lump sum death gratuity
- insurance benefits including enhanced pension on ill health retirement or if redundant from a hospital post
- separate injury benefits scheme providing a pension and lump sum if a GP is unable to work as a result of injury or illness caused by their NHS work.

Salaried service before becoming a GP

If this is more than 10 years it is pensioned separately using the salaried employee method mentioned above. If the pre-GP service is less than 10 years, it is pensioned as part of the GP pension if this produces a better result. The following example shows how this is done.

If a doctor worked for three years in a hospital followed by 37 years as a GP, the GP pension would be increased as follows:

Hospital service	3
GP service	37
Total service	40
Enhancement factor	40/37
GP pension	£21 238 × 40/37 = £22 960
Lump sum	£22 960 × 3 = £68 880

Salaried service after becoming a GP

If this totals less than one whole time year, the income is added to GP superannuable income and pensioned using the GP method.

If it is more than one whole time year, it is pensioned separately using the salaried employee method.

Purchasing extra benefits

Because GPs do not qualify and enter the NHS pension scheme until about age 24, they cannot achieve the maximum permitted service of 40 years in the scheme by age 60, unless they purchase extra benefits. An additional 9% of superannuable income can be used to buy these extra benefits, making a total contribution of 15%, all of which attracts tax relief.

The following options are available to build up a bigger pension and lump sum at retirement:

- *Buying the unreduced lump sum.* This is only necessary for married men with service before 1972, as explained above, and ensures that the lump sum will be three times the pension.

- *Added years.* Buying added years of scheme membership will result in extra benefits in the same format as in the NHS pension scheme generally, i.e. an extra index linked pension and an extra tax free lump sum of three times that pension. Added years also provide additional insurance cover as the added years contract will be honoured in full if the GP dies in service or retires on health grounds before age 60.

- *Additional voluntary contributions/free standing additional voluntary contributions (AVCs/FSAVCs).* Contributions in this case are invested and will provide an extra pension (but not an extra lump sum), the size of which will depend upon:

    - the amount of money invested (up to the 9% limit)

    - the success of the investment

    - annuity (interest) rates prevailing at retirement. The higher the level of interest rates, the bigger the pension (annuity) which can be purchased with the investment fund; and vice versa

    - the amount deducted by the AVC/FSAVC provider by way of commission and administrative charges.

AVCs are an in-house arrangement organized by the NHS scheme through the Equitable Life company. FSAVCs can be purchased through a provider of your choice. As a general rule, AVCs will be better value than FSAVCs because the level of charges is lower. This has been confirmed by recent independent surveys and is also the expressed view of the NHS pension scheme itself. With AVC/FSAVCs, it is only possible for GPs to achieve 38.1 years of service by age 60 whereas by using added years, the maximum entitlement of 40 years service can be reached. GPs cannot forego tax relief on their NHS scheme contributions (see below) if they are contributing to an AVC/FSAVC contract but they can do so if they are purchasing added years.

The advantages and disadvantages of added years and AVCs/FSAVCs are summarized in Box 13.3. FSAVCs generate a commission for the seller, whereas added years and AVCs do not, and care needs to be taken if a financial adviser recommends an FSAVC. The BMA Superannuation Department guidance note entitled *Improving Pension and Lump Sum Benefits* provides further information. If still in doubt, independent financial advice can be obtained from BMA Services Ltd.

Personal pension plans (PPPs)

'Topping up' – using income not taken into account for NHS pension scheme purposes

In this case, the income available for a PPP is the difference between the net Schedule D assessment and the NHS superannuable income in any tax year.

Renouncing tax relief

Because GPs can only claim tax relief on their NHS pension scheme contributions by means of a special extra-statutory concession, they are in the unique position of being able to forego this tax relief but remain in the NHS scheme and pension their income in a PPP as well. In effect, this means that NHS superannuable income may be pensioned twice. This is an attractive option but the higher outgoings involved need to be balanced against the pension benefits eventually accruing.

Spouses' pensions

GPs may contribute towards a PPP for a spouse employed by the practice.

Box 13.3: Added years/AVCs/FSAVCs

Scheme feature	Added years	AVCs	FSAVCs
Contributions	Cannot vary	Variable and flexible	Variable and flexible
Benefit limits	40 years at age 60	Equivalent of 38.1 years at age 60	Equivalent of 38.1 years at age 60
GPs not claiming tax relief on NHS scheme contributions	Available	Not available	Not available
Widows'/ Widowers'* and children's benefits	Available at no extra cost	Available at extra cost	Available at extra cost
Death in service/ ill health benefits	Service usually enhanced	Based on size of fund	Bazed on size of fund
Extra lump sum	Three times extra pension	Not available	Not available
Indexing of pension	Linked to retail prices index	Available with lower pension	Available with lower pension
Tax relief on contributions	Must not exceed 15% of superannuable income	Must not exceed 15% of taxable income	Must not exceed 15% of taxable income
Dependent upon investment returns	No	Yes	Yes
Dependent upon annuity rates at retirement	No	Yes	Yes
Charges and commissions	None	Low	Take care

* Widowers from 6 April 1988

PPPs: taking further advice

The arrangements summarized above are complicated and GPs thinking of using them should be sure to take specialist advice from their accountants or other reputable source. Independent financial advice can be obtained from BMA Services Ltd and, for doctors within the North South Thames regions, specialist taxation and accountancy advice is available from BMA Professional Services Ltd.

Box 13.4: Details of pensions agencies

England and Wales:
NHS Pensions Agency
Hesketh House
200–220 Broadway
Fleetwood, Lancashire
FY7 8LG
Tel: (01253) 774774

Scotland:
Scottish Office Pensions Agency
St Margaret's House
151 London Road
Edinburgh
EH8 7TG
Tel: (0131) 244 3585 or (0131) 556 8400

Northern Ireland:
Health and Personal Social Services
Superannuation Branch (HRD 6)
Waterside House
75 Duke Street
Londonderry
BT47 1FP
Tel: (01504) 319000

---

14 Fundholding

Where to obtain advice and assistance

Any practice considering entry to the fundholding scheme should contact its Health Authority or Health Board.

Further information is available from Henry S and Pickersgill D (eds) (1995) *Making Sense of Fundholding,* Radcliffe Medical Press, Oxford and Pirie A and Kelly-Madden M (1994) *Fundholding: A Practice Guide,* Radcliffe Medical Press, Oxford.

Advisory notes can be obtained from the BMA's General Medical Services Committee. The National Association of Fundholding Practices is also a useful source of advice.

This chapter outlines the basic principles of the fundholding scheme, which was introduced in 1991 as a key element in the Government's NHS changes. It was designed to give GPs 'buying power' in the new internal market. Although entry was restricted initially to a small minority of practices, it was hoped that their purchasing decisions would serve as a stimulus to the internal market.

What is fundholding?

In summary a fundholding practice:

* negotiates a budget with the Health Authority to enable it to purchase a specific range of hospital and community services and to cover the costs of NHS medicines and practice staff
* negotiates contracts with providers for a specific range of hospital care

- has its funds for hospital and community services held by the Health Authority, which pays the providers directly on the practice's behalf when authorized to do so by the practice

- has its budget for prescribing costs held on its behalf by the Health Authority which is debited for the true NHS cost (i.e. basic price less discount) of medicines prescribed

- receives funds to cover a proportion of staff costs

- can provide a limited range of additional, non-general medical services to its own patients and be paid via the fund

- provides monthly reports and an annual statement of accounts to the Health Authority or Health Board

- allows audit of its accounts by the Audit Commission, which should visit the practice at least once every three years

- is allowed to retain any surplus which, after auditing and retention for one year, may be used for health-related projects approved by the Health Authority

- will be reimbursed up to £26 694 (in 1996/97) for additional expenses actually incurred in preparing to be a fundholder and up to £53 952 annually for management expenses incurred whilst actually running the fund.

GP fundholding from April 1996 has taken three forms:

1 *Community fundholding*: a new option for practices with 3000 or more patients (no limit for Scotland and Wales) or for those who are not ready to take on standard fundholding. The scheme will include staff, drugs, diagnostic tests and community health services. It will exclude all hospital treatments (including out-patients).

2 *Standard fundholding*: an extended version of the existing scheme. In addition to existing services, this will include virtually all elective surgery and out-patients services and specialist nursing services. Standard fundholding will be open to practices with least 5000 patients compared with the minimum of 7000 under the current scheme.

3 *Total fundholding (TFH)*: where fundholders in a locality purchase all hospital and community health services for their patients, including accident and emergency services. There are already four pilot projects currently underway (in Bromsgrove, Berkshire, Runcorn and Worth Valley – further details are available from the GMSC office), and a further 44 TFH sites have been approved around the UK all of whom will be evaluated by a university consortium. All of the four initial projects are being evaluated individually.

The NHS Executive has produced a framework and criteria for the evaluation. The 49 sites will cover 2 million of the UK population, and there may be other approved TFH sites but they will not be part of the national evaluation scheme.

Total fundholders do not as yet manage actual budgets as they are still developmental pilot projects. Only fundholding monies can statutorily be devolved to GPFHs so that TFH in whatever form it takes (there are slightly different administrative models) will be accountable for managing the budget but ultimate responsibility will rest with Health Authorities.

Advantages and disadvantages of fundholding

The following are some advantages:

- Collecting the data can in itself be a useful educational exercise
- Fundholding enables GPs to plan and manage more directly the care provided for their patients and to make more direct decisions about how NHS money should be spent
- Fundholders can use savings they make from the fund to improve services for their patients
- Fundholding allows a more flexible approach to managing the practice
- Fundholders are able to transfer money from one element of the fund to another
- The contracting process encourages interaction between NHS bodies which may lead to increased co-operation; for example, close intra-professional relationships between consultants and GPs
- Fundholders can influence directly how hospital and community health services are delivered to their patients.

Some disadvantages include the following:

- Fundholding entails considerable additional work and responsibility for the practice; in particular the preparatory period involves a significant amount of data collection
- There is a risk that the doctor/patient relationship could be adversely influenced; a GP could be perceived as the controller of access to health care, instead of the patient's advocate
- There is a risk of conflict between GPs and hospitals as the NHS internal market becomes increasingly purchase driven. The fundholding

practice occupies a position of influence that is unfamiliar to the secondary care sector

- NHS administrative costs increase, particularly in general practice, but also in hospitals because there are many more purchasers to deal with and substantially more detailed financial and activity reports to provide
- Fundholding can lead to a two-tier delivery of NHS care.

Applying to become a fundholder

Application and assessment procedures vary, but the following account illustrates how health authorities approach these.

- During September and October (i.e. 18–19 months before fundholding status is to be assumed) Health Authorities identify those practices eligible and interested in becoming fundholders and send them the eligibility criteria form. The form requires details of a practice's management arrangements, prescribing policy, computer system and a short statement outlining its reasons for wishing to join the scheme.
- By the end of the following January the Health Authority visits applicants and advises on the suitability of practices.
- By the end of February the Health Authority approves those practices it considers suitable to commence preparatory work.
- By mid-March a plan of how the practice intends to spend the preparatory allowance must be sent to the Health Authority.
- By 31 March, the application form for recognition as a fundholding practice must be completed and received by the Health Authority. It must be signed by all partners in the practice.
- Data collection takes place between 1 April and 30 September of the preparatory year. These data are based on the discharge letters received by the practice and requests for diagnostic tests and direct access services which it has sent to providers.
- Before fundholding status is confirmed, the practice needs to demonstrate that it has the expertise and management structures to run the fund effectively.
- By the end of December (i.e. three months before 'going live') practices must send their Health Authority a purchasing plan which includes a statement of how they satisfy (or propose to satisfy) the assessment criteria and a preliminary plan for the use of the management allowance.

- Successful applicants will be informed by the end of February that they may become fundholders and will receive a budget offer at the same time. A practice must agree the level of fundholding within one month of the offer being made.

The assessment criteria include:

- *list size:* the practice or group of practices must have, or demonstrate that it will have by the start of fundholding, a minimum list size of 5000 (4000 in Scotland) and 3000 in community fundholding practices (there is no list size requirement in the Scottish equivalent of primary care purchasing practices)
- *partnership commitment:* all partners must be in agreement on entry to fundholding
- *managerial support:* the practice must demonstrate that it will be able to manage the fund effectively, efficiently and economically
- *computing support:* the practice must have the necessary computing hardware and software which complies with Health Department specifications (Health Authority grants are available to reimburse costs)
- *data collection:* during the preparatory year practices will have shown that their data collection and analysis is effective
- *purchasing plan:* practices will be asked to produce some form of purchasing plan based on the health needs of their patients within the budgetary constraints.

Preparing for fundholding

Fund management

The fund may be managed by one or more persons, full or part-time. This task may be undertaken by a partner or the practice manager, or the practice may appoint a fund manager. The fund does not have to be managed by an accountant although the practice must have access to accountancy expertise and the partners should be able to understand the accounts.

Staff training

Practice staff will require additional training in various areas, including health needs assessment, negotiating skills and other contracting aspects, computing, business planning, accountancy, financial forecasting and data collection. Part of the preparatory allowance can be used to train staff in skills relevant to fundholding. Computer training costs may be included in software charges and can be claimed from the Health Authority as part of the computer reimbursement.

Computing

Prospective fundholders must acquire sufficient computing facilities. There are several suppliers of software whose systems have Health Department approval. The Health Authority can advise practices on the choice of software. Fundholders are reimbursed by the Health Authority for 100% of the software and associated maintenance and training costs, and 75% of the additional hardware costs, if an approved package is selected and the costs are 'reasonable'. It is advisable to seek the views of other local fundholders about the systems they use.

Changes to the method of purchasing fundholding computer systems

- *Payments*: from 1 April 1996, reimbursement for the purchase of computer systems made through the statement of fees and allowances was replaced by an additional element within the practice fund management allowance (PFMA).
- *Use of funds*: GP fundholders are able to use these sums to purchase, or lease, fundholding computer systems with the prior agreement of the Health Authority. The amount is agreed as part of the practice plan.

The preparatory allowance

An allowance is available during the preparatory year. It can be used to employ staff to collate and retrieve data, to train staff, to buy external advice, to pay for locums whilst partners are preparing for fundholding (up to £4500) and to purchase equipment. (Up to 50% may be spent on equipment.) The fixed standard fundholding preparatory allowance, per fund, is £21 255.

Consortia/grouped practices

Grouped practices

Two or more practices each with list sizes below 7000 may combine to become fundholders. Groups should enter into agreements to apportion the fund, decide how it will be managed and how legal liabilities will be discharged.

Consortia

Practices may form consortia to achieve more negotiating leverage, economies of scale and lower operational costs. This arrangement can enable smaller practices and practices with limited management capacity to participate in the scheme. Each practice/group within a consortium retains responsibility for its budget, even if it is managed centrally.

Scope of the fund

The fund covers four main areas:

- hospital services
- community health services
- prescribed medicines
- practice staff.

Hospital services

The hospital services element covers most outpatient procedures, a defined range of elective inpatient and day case procedures, diagnostic services and direct access services. The fund only covers patients who are registered permanently on the fundholder's list; it excludes temporary residents and includes only those operations and procedures which the Health Department has decided to cover through the fundholding scheme. Therefore, the practice is financially responsible for only those activities that have been initiated or authorized by it, apart from tertiary referrals made by consultants. These must also be paid for from the fund if the practice has been notified of the referral.

The fund does not cover:

- emergency treatment
- obstetrics and genito-urinary medicine
- inpatient stays which do not involve a listed operation or procedure.

There is a £6000 threshold per patient for hospital and community health services above which the Health Authority is liable to pay for treatment for the remainder of the financial year. Prescription costs are not included in this threshold.

Community health services

In April 1993 the hospital and community care component was extended to include:

- district nursing
- health visiting
- chiropody
- dietetics
- all community and outpatient mental health services
- mental health counselling
- health services for people with a learning disability
- referrals made by health visitors and district nurses
- referrals made by social services and other agencies to community nursing services and to learning disabilities services.

Prescribing costs

The fund covers all prescribing on FP10s including drugs and appliances; the £6000 limit does not apply to the prescribing budget.

Practice staff costs

There is no formal guidance to cover the use of the practice staff element of the fund over and above the requirements of the terms of service and statement of fees and allowances. Fundholders must ensure that quality of care to patients is maintained and staff must be appropriately qualified and experienced.

The management allowance

Because managing the fund is an additional task for the practice, fundholders are entitled to a management allowance of up to £53 952 (for 1996/97). This can be used in various ways:

- paying wages to manage the fund
- paying for accountancy, consultancy or other professional services
- purchase of equipment (e.g. computers) – up to 25% of the allowance.

Contracts

There are four basic types of contract.

Block contracts

This is the simplest type: the practice pays an annual fee in instalments to a hospital for access to a specific range of services; for example, pathology or radiography services. This contract may be viewed as funding a given level of activity (known as an indicative volume). At practice level costs must still be attributed (albeit notionally) to individual patients.

Cost and volume contracts

Hospitals receive a sum for a baseline level of activity defined in terms of a predetermined number of treatments or cases; beyond this level funding is on a cost per case basis.

Cost per case contracts

The payment is on a case by case basis, without prior commitment to the volume of cases which might be referred.

Fixed price non attributable contracts

The contract is fixed price in that it is not sensitive in any way to volume or activity. No referrals are recorded in the fundholding software and therefore costs and referrals are not attributable to individual patients. (This means that the £6000 limit per patient cannot apply.) This differs from a block contract where notional costs are always attributed to individual patients. Since 1993 this type has applied to community services.

Contracting with non-NHS providers

Fundholders may contract with private providers of specialist services if they have been allocated a provider number by the Health Authority. Fundholders should ensure that the professional staff providing care are properly qualified. Fundholders should note that contracts with non-NHS bodies are legally binding on the practice. (Since 1993/94 community staff contracts may only be made with current NHS providers.)

Special referral arrangements

Practices may arrange with NHS providers for consultants to hold NHS sessions in their surgery premises. Alternatively, fundholders may employ directly the services of a consultant (or another practitioner such as a physiotherapist) on a private basis if this is less costly, or perhaps more convenient, than an outpatient referral to an NHS hospital. Such practitioners could be employed on the practice premises or elsewhere. In these circumstances, as with GPs acting in a private capacity, the patient remains an NHS patient but the consultant or practitioner is working in a private capacity and cannot count this work as an NHS session.

The extension of services provided by fundholders

Since April 1993 fundholders have been able to offer a limited range of services (e.g. vasectomies, varicose vein surgery, blood counts, upper gastrointestinal endoscopy, colposcopy and audiometry) covered by the scheme to their own patients, over and above those services provided within general medical services, and may make an appropriate charge on the fund for these. These new arrangements bar limited companies from being used by fundholders to provide services to patients.

Managing the fund

It is the responsibility of the fundholder to ensure that the fund allocated to them is managed 'efficiently and effectively'.

Overspending

The Health Authority receives an overall cash limited financial allocation for all purchasers in its region; therefore a fundholder's fund is acquired at the expense of Health Authority purchasers because they no longer have to purchase those services covered by the fund on behalf of fundholders' patients.

An overspend resulting from poor management may lead to a practice losing its fundholding status. Where overspends occur, additional funding has to be provided by Health Authorities to meet the fundholder's commitments so that services to patients are not interrupted. In some circumstances a Health Authority may consider that an overspend is due to factors outside the control of the fundholder and not therefore due to mismanagement; for example, if the overspend is caused by:

- an unanticipated significant increase in list size
- an unanticipated significant increase in the number of high cost patients on the practice list (especially if they need high cost drugs)
- a serious epidemic
- errors or discrepancies in either the data or the costs used by the Health Authority as the basis for setting the level of the fund.

The 1993 regulations include powers to enable Health Authorities to recover misapplied sums through the civil courts. The Health Department has assured the BMA that it has no intention of using the 'misapplication' regulation to initiate proceedings against any fundholding practice which *inadvertently* overspends on its funds on activities covered by NHS Acts.

Underspending and use of savings

Underspending may be due to various circumstances:

- fundholders may make savings in a particular area: for example, they may adopt a new prescribing policy and make savings on this component of the fund
- fundholders may obtain unplanned savings: for example, they expect (and plan for) a higher level of service than their patients actually require
- the original level of the fund from the Health Authority may have been inaccurate.

If the underspending is due to the Health Authority setting the level of the fund too high, the fundholder is permitted to keep the unspent money as savings. However, the level will obviously be reviewed in subsequent years. Fundholders cannot spend savings until they have been officially audited. They may be carried over for up to four years. Savings can be spent on activities covered by the fund, or for one or more of the following purposes (subject to Health Authority approval):

- purchasing materials or equipment which:
  - can be used for the treatment of patients in the practice
  - enhance the comfort or convenience of patients
  - enable the practice to be managed more effectively and efficiently

- purchasing of materials or equipment relating to health education
- improving the practice premises or its furnishings and fitting.

Fundholders will only be able to fund practice staff posts for the period it takes to use up the sum allocated from the savings; therefore staff may have to be appointed on a temporary basis.

The Health Authority is responsible for ensuring the fundholders' proposed use of savings comply with the fundholding regulations.

15 Medical Politics: how GPs are represented

Like their counterparts in other branches of the medical profession, GPs belong to a wide variety of representational, professional and learned bodies, and pressure groups. Some cater for the entire profession such as the General Medical Council, BMA, the medical defence organizations and the Royal Society of Medicine; whereas others serve the interests of a minority, for example the Overseas Doctors Association, Dispensing Doctors Association and the National Association of Fundholding Practices. This chapter explains how the interests of all GPs are collectively represented through their own democratic machinery, which is based on the links between LMCs and the BMA's GMSC.

Because it is such a well-established profession, medicine enjoys a large measure of self government in its relationship to the State. This self government has generated a variety of medico-political institutions, including those which enable doctors to be represented on bodies concerned with running of the NHS. In particular, NHS GPs are represented by a national body, the GMSC, and a network of 126 LMCs.

Background

The origins of the GMSC and the LMCs date back to 1913, when a publicly funded health service (albeit restricted to providing GP services to a minority of the adult population) was first introduced by Lloyd George's National Insurance Act. When this legislation was proposed it made no provision for GPs to be involved in the running of the new state health service. However, the BMA was determined that the profession should have a voice and its efforts ensured that locally elected committees of GPs (LMCs) were statutorily recognized in the Act as the democratic voice of GPs in each locality. Thus the Act required Local Insurance Committees (the forerunners of NHS Executive Councils, Family Practitioner Committees (FPCs) and latterly FHSAs), whose task was to run this new health insurance scheme, to consult through the LMC all GPs participating in the new health service on many administrative and professional matters.

Once LMCs were established, the BMA formed a national committee based on them to represent GPs' interests in negotiations with government. This committee, the Insurance Acts Committee, the forerunner of the GMSC, was recognized by government as the democratic voice of GPs.

The Liberal Government agreed to these arrangements for representing GPs because the success of its health insurance scheme depended on the willing co-operation of GPs. Although the profession ostensibly supported the concept of a state medical scheme it was opposed to it being provided by salaried doctors. It believed that if GPs' independent contractor status was replaced by a salaried service this would undermine their freedom to practise without state interference and affect adversely patient care. GPs and their representatives suspected that government would attempt to influence their day-to-day care of patients.

Commitment to the independent contractor status remains a guiding principle of the GMSC. Had it not been for the tenacity of its forerunner (the Insurance Acts Committee) on this crucial issue, GPs could have been unwillingly sucked into a salaried service (as were their hospital colleagues in 1948). The well-tested and proven value of the contract for service with local insurance committees led to this type of contract continuing and developing within the NHS following its inception in 1948. The local insurance committees recognized that this contract worked well and sought successfully to preserve it in the new NHS structure.

Health Authorities recognize LMCs

LMCs must be formally recognized by Health Authorities in order to carry out their statutory functions and raise funds through the statutory levy for their day-to-day operation. This statutory recognition of the LMC has parallels elsewhere in the public sector; legislation enacted in the 1940s to nationalize public utilities and major industries explicitly recognized trade unions and professional associations for negotiating and consultative purposes. The statutory recognition accorded to LMCs was granted almost 40 years earlier; the earliest example in the UK of an organization being recognized by statute to represent those providing a publicly funded service.

Three types of functions and duties of LMCs derive from their recognition by Health Authorities:

- those based on the 'partnership principle' (originating in 1911): on many key issues LMCs and Health Authorities determine jointly what policies and actions should be implemented. This local recognition and representation ensures the efficient provision of general medical services, enabling Health Authorities to draw upon the goodwill and experience of local GPs. The process of consultation also ensures that the terms of service (negotiated centrally by the GMSC and Health Department) are fairly and reasonably applied locally

- those concerned with administering the GP contract. Health Authorities are obliged to consult LMCs on many issues; this is evident in the regulations governing NHS general medical services, GPs' terms of service and the statement of fees and allowances. The LMC also plays an important role in both the complaints procedure and the investigation of certain matters relating to professional conduct

- those concerned with representing GPs as a whole.

LMCs also provide many other services for their GP constituents which vary according to local 'custom and practice'. These include handling local ethical problems, representing GPs in relations with bodies and organizations outside the NHS, and promoting the standing of general practice both in the media and among the public generally. To this end many LMCs have established close ties with MPs, local councillors, community health councils, and other professions such as nursing, health visiting and social work.

Other health service bodies

The LMC also serves as a point of reference for other NHS bodies seeking GPs' views; a perusal of LMC activities shows that this is a large part of their work. Although GPs are no longer represented, as of right, on Health Authorities, a few continue to serve on these bodies. In some areas, LMCs appoint doctors to serve on regional medical advisory committees, regional GP advisory subcommittees, purchasing advisory bodies, district medical advisory committees (where these are established), and also on variously named district medical liaison/executive committees, the regional GP subcommittees for postgraduate medical education, and many other *ad hoc* committees and working groups (clinical and administrative) at regional, district and local levels. LMCs are consulted when GPs are appointed to many offices and posts, and they play an active part in advising their local health authorities on a range of policy matters, including recently, and most importantly, the commissioning of secondary care. In short, LMCs have a continuing dialogue with other parts of the NHS. They also become involved in many other issues affecting GPs locally: examples include clinical assistant and hospital practitioner grade posts, GP hospitals and units, GP beds, and access to diagnostic facilities.

LMCs medico-political functions

The LMC is an independent self-financing body with statutory functions (as distinct from a state-funded statutory body). Its independent status allows it to exercise medico-political and statutory functions. This duality of roles is unique and contributes to its strength. The statutory functions are mostly concerned with protecting the interests of individual GPs in relation to their contract, and also with the continuing consultations and negotiations between LMCs and Health Authorities. On the other hand, the medico-political functions are concerned primarily with the collective interests of GPs as a group, and they operate through a quite separate channel consisting of the annual conference of LMC representatives and the GMSC.

In some areas, regional committees of LMCs provide a forum for discussing supra-district problems and exchanging ideas and experience. In these circumstances regional local medical committees provide an important link with NHSE regional offices.

GMSC

The GMSC is a BMA committee with authority to deal with all matters affecting NHS GPs. It represents all GPs in Great Britain, whether or not they are members of the BMA (in fact over 70% are members).

The committee is recognized as the sole negotiating body for general practice by the Health Department and is represented in negotiations with ministers and civil servants by a team of five GPs who draw upon their day-to-day experience of general practice and are assisted by full-time expert advisers. The team is supplemented by other GMSC members and legal, accountancy and other specialist advice as and when necessary.

The GMSC has 83 members, of whom 44 are directly elected representatives of LMCs. It meets monthly and much of its work is done by subcommittees and task groups (*see* Box 15.1). It is represented on most national bodies concerned with health, providing an essential medical input which is firmly rooted in the day-to-day experience of general practice (*see* Box 15.2). The Welsh and Scottish GMSCs are subcommittees of the national GMSC, but have autonomy on NHS matters exclusive to their countries. The Northern Ireland GMSC is autonomous of the GMSC but has close working relations with it.

Box 15.1: The GMSC subcommittees' activities

Scottish GMSC
- GPs working in the NHS in Scotland: negotiates directly with the Scottish Home and Health Department

Welsh GMSC
- GPs working in the NHS in Wales: negotiates directly with the Welsh Office

General purposes subcommittee
- all matters referred to it by the GMSC; also considers relationships between GPs and colleagues in other health professions

Education and audit subcommittee
- all matters relating to professional audit, vocational training, undergraduate and continuing education for GPs

Information management and technology subcommittee
- the development and application of computers in general practice

Commissioning of care subcommittee
- advises on GP involvement in the commissioning process

Fundholding subcommittee
- represents the interests of fundholding GPs

Hospital and special services subcommittee
- terms of service and contractual arrangements of GPs working in hospitals: obstetric care, minor surgery, child health surveillance, contraceptive services, cervical cytology and health promotion

Prescribing subcommittee
- prescribing and the supply of medicines

Rural practice subcommittee
- general practice in rural areas, including GP dispensing

Statute and regulations subcommittee
- any NHS Acts, statutory instruments and other parliamentary legislation relevant to NHS general practice

continued opposite

Box 15.1: *continued*

Registrars subcommittee
- represents the interests of GP vocational trainees

Task groups on
- practice premises
- mental health services
- medical workforce
- GMSC constitution
- GMSC business

Box 15.2: GMSC representation on outside bodies

Advisory Committee on Borderline Substances
Advisory Committee on Cervical Screening
Advisory Committee on NHS Drugs
Advisory Group on Medical Education, Training and Staffing
Association of Medical Secretaries, Practice Administrators
    and Receptionists

BMA/Association of British Pharmaceutical Industry Liaison
    Committee
BMA/Overseas Doctors Association Working Party
BMA/Royal College of Nursing Liaison Committee
BMA/Royal Pharmaceutical Society of Great Britain Liaison
    Committee

Chief Executive/Chief Medical Officers Working Group
Chief Executive Working Group on Information Management
    and Technology
Child Health Computing Committee
Child Health Informatics Consortium
Churches Council for Health and Healing
Clinical Standards Advisory Group
Committee of Postgraduate Medical Deans
Committee on Standards of Data Extraction

Family Planning Association, Medical Advisory Group

continued overleaf

Box 15.2: *continued*

General Dental Services Committee
General Medical Council: Medical Assessors
GP Systems Accreditation Group

Health Service Commissioner: Professional Advisers

Joint Committee on Postgraduate Training for General Practice
Joint Consultants Committee

Medical Information Group
Medical Practices Committee

National Cervical Screening Programme Co-ordinating Network
New NHS Number Project Board
NHS Centre for Coding and Classification Supervisory Board
NHS Tribunal: Panel of Medical Practitioners

Overseas Accreditation Panel

Prescription Pricing Authority
Public Health Laboratory Service Board

Royal College of General Practitioners Council
Royal College of General Practitioners Education Committee
Royal College of General Practitioners Liaison Committee

Service Committees and Tribunal Regulations: Medical
    Advisory Committees
Standing Committee on Postgraduate Medical Education
Standing Medical Advisory Committee
Strategic Advisory Group for Clinical IM&T Systems
Summative Assessment Advisory Panel

UK Central Committee for Nursing, Midwifery and
    Health Visiting
Union of European GPs (UEMO)

The GMSC's policy-making procedures operate on an annual cycle. It sends all GPs an annual report of its work in March. Individual GPs can influence policy through their LMCs which consider the report and submit motions to the annual conference of LMC representatives held in June. This conference, comprising more than 300 GPs appointed by LMCs, is the profession's principal policy-making body. Those motions which are approved by the conference are referred to the GMSC to implement. This democratic process gives credibility to the GMSC's day-to-day activities as the representative voice of all NHS GPs.

This description of the LMC conference/GMSC structure shows how GPs have exercised 'self-government' through their LMCs. Every part of the UK has at least one spokesperson on the GMSC; a doctor working in practice who can represent its problems and express its views on issues affecting negotiations for GPs as a whole.

Negotiations with government

There is a regular cycle of meetings between the GMSC negotiating team and a team of Health Department officials, and these are supplemented by many other meetings to deal with specific matters. Indeed, contact between the GMSC secretariat and the Health Department is normally as frequent as several times each working day; thus there is a continuing dialogue between the two sides. Over the years negotiations have covered a wide range of issues. In practice, the satisfactory completion of negotiations only occasionally results in major amendments to the Red Book and, even more rarely, amendments to the legal framework of general practice, the NHS regulations (which include the GP's terms of service). It is important to note that the Red Book, although technically part of the NHS regulations, can be amended without parliamentary approval, whereas because the NHS regulations themselves are parliamentary enactments they require parliamentary approval to amend their provisions.

General medical services defence fund

This representative system involves a considerable expenditure of time and money, and the Defence Fund (first established in 1913) is the main source of funds for running it. The term 'defence' may appear to be a misnomer if narrowly defined to apply only to some form of direct action against Government (e.g. the collection of undated resignations from the NHS);

however, the GMSC's work together with that of its subcommittees and working groups, is aimed at defending GPs' interests both collectively and individually, even though the profession may not be engaged in a confrontation with Government on any specific issue. All this activity costs money; it could be described as the price the profession has to pay for 'self-government'.

Statutory and voluntary levies

Most of the income for the defence fund comes from voluntary contributions raised by LMCs from their constituent GPs. This voluntary levy is quite distinct from the statutory levy; the latter may be used only 'for defraying the administrative expenses of the LMC, including travelling and subsistence allowances payable to its members'. Although the legislation allows LMCs (in England and Wales only) to make a compulsory statutory levy on every GP to meet these specific expenses, not all LMCs choose to do so. Each LMC determines for itself whether to raise its funds from either the voluntary levy or both the voluntary and statutory levies.

16 Entering General Practice: The GP Vocational Training Scheme

Before 1981, when vocational training for general practice became mandatory, any fully registered medical practitioner could apply to fill a GP vacancy as a partner or single-handed practitioner. However, a doctor without previous GP experience was rarely admitted to an FPC medical list. Long before vocational training became compulsory, most doctors wishing to become GPs were already extending their obligatory one year pre-registration hospital training by gaining further hospital experience, as well as filling traineeships, or sometimes assistantships, before joining a practice.

The vocational training regulations

These regulations govern entry to general practice; all doctors applying to become NHS GP principals, whether single-handed or in partnership, have to show that they have acquired a specified range of postgraduate experience. Currently they do not apply to doctors who work as:

- whole-time practitioners in private general practice
- assistants in NHS general practice
- restricted services principals in the NHS; that is providing services which are limited to child health surveillance, contraceptive services, maternity medical services, minor surgery services, or some combination of these
- deputies for commercial deputizing services.

Other doctors may be exempt because:

- they were already GP principals on 15 February 1981 when the regulations first applied (these doctors remain permanently exempt and if they resign and subsequently return to general practice this exemption is preserved)
- they have been engaged on comparable duties in the armed forces to those of general practice.

The regulations prescribe what clinical experience has to be acquired to obtain the 'certificate of prescribed experience' issued by the Joint Committee on Postgraduate Training for General Practice (JCPTGP). The Medical Practices Committee (MPC) which ultimately determines whether a vacancy (in a partnership or single-handed) should be filled, and who should fill it, requires all applications for a principalship to be supported by a JCPTGP certificate.

Because the UK is required to implement a European directive on GP vocational training all doctors working in general practice are required to satisfy the vocational training regulations.

From 1 January 1994, doctors will need to have from the JCPTGP either:

- a certificate of prescribed experience issued on completion of vocational training, or
- a certificate of equivalent experience.

Certain categories of doctors are, however, exempt from the provisions of the directive by possessing an 'acquired right' to practise. In the United Kingdom the doctors who have been identified as entitled to an acquired right are:

- all doctors practising as principals in general practice on 31 December 1994

- all doctors who are eligible to become principals under the NHS (Vocational Training) Regulations by virtue of the fact that they were principals in general practice on or after 15 February 1981 or, if employed in the armed services, in possession of a statement of exemption from the director general of medical services, or in possession of a certificate of prescribed/equivalent experience issued by the JCPTGP

- any doctor who has worked as an assistant (including on the retainer scheme) or deputy (including locum) in the UK on either 10 separate days in the ten years ending 31 December 1994, has an acquired right to work in either of these capacities (but not as a principal).

What is 'prescribed experience'?

This requires three years' training comprising:

- at least one year as a GP registrar

- at least one year comprising two or more hospital appointments of at least six months each in two or more of these specialties: accident and emergency medicine or general surgery, general medicine, geriatrics, obstetrics and/or gynaecology, paediatrics, psychiatry. The entire hospital 'leg' of the vocational training may be confined to any two of these specialties

- alternatively any remaining period (up to one year) may be spent on one or more of a wider range of hospital or community medicine posts or in a GP training practice.

These posts must be 'educationally approved' which means being approved by the Royal College or Faculty relevant to each specialty, and being selected by a regional postgraduate education committee as suitable for GP vocational training.

GP trainers (i.e. the approval of GP training posts) are selected by regional committees for postgraduate medical education, advised by their general practice subcommittees.

Vocational GP registrars have to obtain a 'statement of satisfactory completion' for each separate appointment they have filled and present these to the JCPTGP.

The formal definition of 'satisfactory completion' in Box 16.1 makes no reference to any requirement that GP registrars should demonstrate the knowledge and skills they have acquired. However, legal advice has confirmed that satisfactory completion indicates a satisfactory level of competence, according to the assessment of the person signing the statement

---

Box 16.1:

'Satisfactory completion' of a period of training is defined as completing it "in such a manner as to have acquired the medical experience which may reasonably be expected from training of that duration in that employment".

---

of satisfactory completion, and this view has been jointly endorsed by the chairmen of the GMSC, the JCPTGP and the Council of the RCGP. Thus doctors completing vocational training for general practice are expected to have achieved a satisfactory standard of competence and performance.

The joint committee formally introduced from September 1996 a process of summative assessment to guarantee that an appropriate standard has been achieved. This will be given a regulatory framework by September 1997 as indicated in the Government's white paper *Primary Care: Delivering the Future.*

The BMA's General Medical Services Committee has expressed concern about the flawed method of implementation of summative assessment, including its introduction mid-way through many GP registrars' training, and the undue haste of implementation without adequate funding. At the time of writing, the GMSC is pursuing the question of additional resources with the health department.

Equivalent experience

Other kinds of clinical experience which do not necessarily fulfil the criteria of prescribed experience may count as 'equivalent' to prescribed experience; examples include:

• posts occupied on a less than half-time basis or for less than six months

• experience gained outside the UK

• 'electives'

• experience gained in occupational health.

If the JCPTGP is satisfied that a doctor's overall experience is indeed equivalent to that prescribed by the regulations it issues a certificate of equivalent experience, which has the same standing as a 'prescribed' experience certificate.

Equivalent experience provides a way of satisfying the regulations other than by conventional vocational training. However, the experience gained must equate in educational terms with that prescribed in the regulations; the standardized programme of training and its permitted variations. The difficulties of equating like with like are considerable and the JCPTGP has developed a substantial body of case law which enables it to judge whether a particular range of experience satisfies the criteria. A doctor has a right to appeal to the Secretary of State against the JCPTGP's refusal to issue a certificate of prescribed or equivalent experience.

Vocational training schemes

Normally, full vocational training involves a three-year structured scheme which is usually undertaken immediately after GMC registration. Two of these three years are normally spent in Senior House Officer (SHO) posts and the other in a training practice.

Most GP registrars do their training within a three-year structured scheme organized by regional postgraduate medical education committees. The structured scheme provides a series of rotations in hospital posts and a training practice or practices. Its main advantage is that trainees do not have to find and apply for a succession of posts; they therefore enjoy a greater security of tenure and can plan their lives around the three years of training. The posts on the rotation will be approved educationally and there should be fewer problems in obtaining time off to attend weekly day or half-day release courses.

The other alternative is the self-constructed training programme which can offer greater flexibility in the type and location of hospital posts. This arrangement may be particularly beneficial for doctors who are undecided about their careers and want to keep their options open. The main disadvantage is that they have to compete for a series of posts.

Part-time training

The vocational training regulations allow part-time employment in approved training posts to qualify as prescribed experience, provided the overall length of training is extended proportionately. Part-time is not restricted to half-time employment; less than half-time training may be aggregated to count towards equivalent experience.

Box 16.2: GP registrar's allowances and direct reimbursement

- removal and relocation expenses: these are extensive and complex and based on the NHS General Whitley Council conditions of service
- travelling expenses
- interview expenses ,
- payment during sickness
- maternity leave payments
- expenses for postgraduate examinations

Full details of all these payments are in paragraph 38 of the Red Book.

A model contract for GP registrars

The details of a GP registrar's employment contract are not governed by the vocational training regulations, which pay no regard to hours of duty and holiday arrangements. These and other matters should be agreed before the traineeship in general practice starts and encapsulated in a written employment contract. A model contract is available to BMA members from their local office. However, the trainee's salary and a range of specific allowances and direct reimbursements (particularly those relating to removal expenses) are specified in the Red Book (*see* Box 16.2) and the trainer does not exercise any discretion in relation to these payment. The trainee's salary is fixed by reference to his or her other previous hospital posts. Thus the salary is therefore substantially higher for a former registrar than for someone who was previously an SHO. A trainer cannot pay a GP registrar more than the appropriate salary specified in the Red Book.

Payments made to the GP trainer

The following are paid to trainers when they employ GP registrars:

- a training grant (an allowance for the additional work and costs incurred by employing a trainee)

- reimbursement of the employer's share of the trainee's NI contributions (the GP registrar pays the employee's share)
- a car or motor vehicle allowance, if the practice needs an additional vehicle for the GP registrar
- the cost of installing an extra telephone at the surgery and a telephone at the trainee's residence
- the rental charge for a telephone at the GP registrar's residence (provided the trainee is responsible for paying it) and the cost of installation and rental charge for a bedroom telephone extension at the GP registrar's home, if both the complying authority and trainer are satisfied that it is necessary
- the trainee's salary which is related to the basic salary in the previous NHS hospital post
- reimbursement of the trainee's medical defence organization subscription or premium costs, less any costs which would have been incurred if they had taken out the basic subscription ('additional cover') payable by hospital doctors. The trainer must have evidence of the GP registrar's subscription or premium being paid. The reimbursement may be paid in one lump sum or in monthly instalments to reflect the GP registrar's arrangements for paying the subscription and length of service with the trainer.

The trainer is responsible for administering the GP registrar's NIC and PAYE.

Appendix 1: Local BMA Offices and Staff

England

Bristol

4th Floor
Centre Gate
Colston Avenue
Bristol BS1 4TR
Tel: 0117 922 7645
Fax: 0117 925 2494

Cambridge

10 Downing Street
Cambridge CB2 3DS
Tel: 01223 364539
Fax: 01223 464743

Exeter

Portland House
Langbrook Street
Exeter EX4 6AB
Tel: 01392 276661

Mersey
(includes Isle of Man)

35 Seymour Terrace
Seymour Street
Liverpool L3 5PE
Tel: 0151 709 5660
Fax: 0151 709 5376

North East

First Floor
Holland Park C
Holland Drive
Fenham Barracks
Newcastle NE2 4LD
Tel: 0191 261 7131
Fax: 0191 261 6203

North Thames	BMA House Tavistock Square London WC1H 9JP Tel: 0171 388 8296 Fax: 0171 383 6911
North West	Bartree House 460 Palatine Road Northenden Manchester M22 4DJ Tel: 0161 945 8989 Fax: 0161 945 5045
Oxford	Cranbrook House 287 Banbury Road Summertown Oxford OX2 7JF Tel: 01865 559621 Fax: 01865 558082
South Thames	Venture House 15 High Street Purley Surrey CR8 2XA Tel: 0181 660 5558 Fax: 0181 668 0117
Trent	301 Glossop Road Sheffield S10 2HL Tel: 0114 272 1705 Fax: 0114 275 1686
West Midlands	36 Harborne Road Edgbaston Birmingham B15 3AJ Tel: 0121 456 1402 Fax: 0121 456 3439
Winchester (includes Channel Islands)	Star Lane House Staple Gardens Winchester SO23 8SR Tel: 01962 856760 Fax: 01962 856761

Yorkshire

Gladstone House
Redvers Close
Lawnswood Business Park
Leeds LS16 6SS
Tel: 0113 230 4417
Fax: 0113 230 6144

Scotland

South East Scotland

3 Hill Place
Edinburgh EH8 9EQ
Tel: 0131 662 4820
Fax: 0131 667 6933

West of Scotland

2 Woodside Place
Glasgow G3 7QF
Tel: 0141 332 1862
Fax: 0141 332 2259

North of Scotland

56 Queen's Street
Aberdeen AB1 6YE
Tel: 01224 323311
Fax: 01224 322723

Wales

1 Cleeve House
Cardiff Business Park
Llanishen
Cardiff CF4 5GJ
Tel: 01222 766277
Fax: 01222 766162

Northern Ireland

61 Malone Road
Belfast BT9 6SA
Tel: 01232 663272
Fax: 01232 666318

Appendix 2: BMA Professional Services Ltd

London

BMA House
Tavistock Square
London WC1H 9JP
Tel: 0171 383 6743
Fax: 0171 383 6813

South Thames

Croudace House
97 Godstone Road
Caterham
Surrey CR3 6XQ
Tel: 01883 331215
Fax: 01883 331216

North Thames

York House
Empire Way
Wembley
Middlesex HA9 0PA
Tel: 0181 900 0444
Fax: 0181 903 6185

Trent

Rodney House
Castle Gate
Nottingham NG1 7AW
Tel: 0115 948 0788
Fax: 0115 948 0787

Appendix 3: BMA Services Ltd

Aberdeen	56 Queens Road Aberdeen AB15 4YE Tel: 01224 323311
Belfast	Second and Third Floor 102 Lisburn Road Belfast BT9 6AG Tel: 01232 664609
Birmingham	Maybrook House Queensway Halesowen Birmingham B63 4AH Tel: 0121 585 6474
Bristol	25 Osprey Court Hawkfield Business Park Whitchurch Bristol BS14 0BB Tel: 0117 964 0777
Cardiff	Unit 15 Lambourne Crescent Cardiff Business Park Cardiff CF4 5GG Tel: 01222 766988
Dartford	Instone House Instone Road Dartford Kent DA1 2AG Tel: 01322 272270
Edinburgh	Stanhope House 12 Stanhope Place Edinburgh EH12 5HH Tel: 0131 313 0210

Exeter	Third Floor Portland House Longbrook Street Exeter EX4 6AB Tel: 01392 422456
Glasgow	Breckenridge House 274 Sauchiehall Street Glasgow G2 3EH Tel: 0141 332 1862
Leeds	Gladstone House Redvers Close Lawnswood Business Park Leeds LS16 6UU Tel: 0113 230 6100
Leicester	Premier House 29 Rutland Street Leicester LE1 1RE Tel: 0116 265 0354
Liverpool	35 Seymour Terrace Seymour Street Liverpool L3 5PE Tel: 0151 709 3599
Manchester	Bartree House 460 Palatine Road Northenden Manchester M22 4DJ Tel: 0161 945 5445
Newcastle	Holland Park C Holland Drive Fenham Barracks Newcastle NE2 4LD Tel: 0191 261 9661
Nottingham	Huntingdon House 278–280 Huntingdon Street Nottingham NG1 3LY Tel: 0115 952 4333
Sheffield	305 Glossop Road Sheffield S10 2HL Tel: 0114 279 7813

Uxbridge

3 The Grand Union Office Park
Packet Boat Lane
Uxbridge
Middlesex UB8 2GH
Tel: 01895 850350

North London

Bartholomew Court
60–61 High Street
Waltham Cross
Herts EN8 7DD
Tel: 01992 638121

For general insurance enquiries, the Free Quoteline number is 0500 181 099. This office is based at Colchester.

Index